The Chronically Limited Elderly

The Case for a National Policy for In-Home and Supportive Community-Based Services

The Chronically Limited Elderly

The Case for a National Policy for In-Home and Supportive Community-Based Services

Howard A. Palley, PhD, and Julianne S. Oktay, PhD

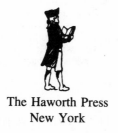

The Haworth Press
New York

The Chronically Limited Elderly: The Case for a National Policy for In-Home and Supportive Community-Based Services has also been published as *Home Health Care Services Quarterly*, Volume 4, Number 2, Summer 1983.

The Haworth Press, Inc., 28 East 22 Street, New York, NY 10010

Library of Congress Cataloging in Publication Data
Main entry under title:

The chronically limited elderly.

"Has also been published as Home health care services quarterly, volume 4, number 2, summer 1983"—T.p. verso.
    Includes bibliographical references.
    1. Community health services for the aged—Government policy—United States.
2. Aged—Home care—Government policy—United States. 3. Aged—Services for—Government policy—United States. 4. Aged—United States—Family relationships. I. Palley, Howard A. II. Oktay, Julianne S. [DNLM: 1. Health services for the aged. 2. Chronic disease—In old age. 3. Home care services. 4. Public policy—United States.
WT 500 C557]
RA564.8.C48   1983   362.6'3   83-10686
ISBN 0-86656-236-2

The Chronically Limited Elderly
The Case for a National Policy for In-Home and Supportive Community-Based Services

Home Health Care Services Quarterly
Volume 4, Number 2

CONTENTS

SECTION III
IN-HOME SERVICES AND THE COMMUNITY-BASED
NETWORK OF SERVICES:
THE STATUS OF CURRENT PROGRAMS AND A REVIEW
AND CRITIQUE OF LEGISLATIVE PROPOSALS

SECTION IV
INTERNATIONAL POLICY CONSIDERATIONS REGARDING
IN-HOME SERVICES FOR THE FRAIL ELDERLY

JANET E. STARR, BS. *Executive Director, Home Care Association of New York State, Inc., Syracuse, New York*

MONNICA C. STEWART, MB, BS, D(Obst), RCOG, *Community Medicine Physician, City and East London Area Health Authority, London, United Kingdom*

ANN-MARIE THOM, *Executive Director, Visiting Nurse Association of New York, New York, New York*

PATRICIA THOMAS, *Executive Director, Visiting Homemakers Association, Toronto, Ontario, Canada*

THOMAS R. WILLEMAIN, PhD, *Associate Professor of Public Policy, John F. Kennedy School of Government, Harvard University, Cambridge, Massachusetts; Senior Research Associate, University Health Policy Consortium, Brandeis University, Waltham, Massachusetts*

JUDITH LA VOR WILLIAMS, *Florence Heller School for Advanced Studies in Social Welfare, Brandeis University, Waltham, Massachusetts*

Acknowledgments

Much of the initial impetus for this study occurred when the authors were co-directors of the National Association of Social Worker's Policy Research Network Project on Family Policy With Respect to Services for the Chronically-Ill Elderly (1980-1981). Work on this project engaged our thinking and focused our concerns. We are grateful to Ms. Susan Rees and Mr. Alfonso Gonzalez of NASW for their encouragement of our efforts. We also appreciate the editorial advice of Ms. Brahna Trager, Dr. Laura Reif, and Dr. Nancy Humphreys.

We would like to thank Sharon Morgan, Gwen Young, and Virginia Peggs for their help in typing innumerable drafts of the manuscript. Also, Assistant Dean Lily Gold, University of Maryland, School of Social Work and Community Planning, was very helpful in facilitating the typing and reproduction of the manuscript. We are forever grateful for her support and help in overcoming the difficulties involved in the production process.

Last, but not least, we also would like to thank our respective spouses, Marian L. Palley and Erol Oktay for their forbearance and encouragement.

Howard A. Palley, PhD
Julianne S. Oktay, PhD
School of Social Work and Community Planning
University of Maryland

SECTION I

THE FAMILY, THE ELDERLY, AND NATIONAL LONG-TERM CARE POLICY

Chapter 1

In-Home and Other Supportive Community-Based Services for the Chronically Limited Elderly: Problems, Prospects, and Proposals

The main goal of this book is to stress the need for a clear national policy designed to provide improved home health and other in-home services for the chronically limited elderly and their families within a comprehensive system of community-based health and social services. This national policy should have as its goal the provision of accessible, comprehensive, and quality health and social support services in the community. A major theme of this volume is that such policy must be developed, funded, and be administratively accountable at the national level. Standards of quality of services, criteria of need, and capital funding support all require a primary role by the national government in the development of such a system. A second main theme which runs throughout the volume is the vital support role of the family. One goal of a national policy focused on provision of in-home services and other supportive community-based services would be to reinforce the efforts of family caregivers and to relieve stress on such family members "coping" with the homebound frail elderly.

In developing this policy perspective, we do not attempt to develop a model "delivery system" for in-home and other community-based services to the frail elderly. In reflecting on other national experiences, we believe that home care for the frail elderly encompassing home health care and in-home social care—as well as supportive community-based services—should be considered neither as a subset of services in the general field of aging, nor as a part of a continuum of social services to families. Home-based care in other national experiences (Denmark, Germany, Sweden, and

Canada) is usually a fusion of in-home health care and social care services. Such services are in part administratively under the health care system and in part under personal social service systems—the mechanisms of integration differ in different national experiences.

The national policy regarding home-based care and other supportive community-based services which we discuss would primarily target on the elderly. It should ideally be available for other chronically limited groups as well.

The Organization of the Study

Following this introductory chapter, the book is divided into four sections, each analyzing the problem at a different level. In the first section, "The Family, the Elderly, and National Long-Term Care Policy," we focus on the health and social problems of the elderly, the role of the family, and the need for a national family policy perspective. In Chapter 2, we begin with a discussion of the growth of the elderly population. We also show how this growth results in increased numbers of chronically ill. Finally, we explore the family life of the elderly, and how it is affected by health problems. Current trends in family life, such as low birth rates, high divorce rates, and high proportions of women in the work force, are discussed as they may be expected to impact on the family's continued ability to provide care for elderly relatives who become ill or disabled.

Chapter 3 moves to a discussion of national family policy. It indicates that current programs which do provide in-home and other community-based services for the chronically limited elderly place little emphasis on the impact of such long-term care policy on the family's role. Such community-based programs stress service for *acute* illness, while the elderly are more likely to have *chronic* health problems which require a variety of community-based long-term care services. On a national basis, such in-home and other community-based services which are available often vary greatly in quality, availability, and program integration. In addition, current long-term care policy emphasizes an institutional nursing home approach rather than community-based services. Finally, we elaborate upon the substantial gap between the needs of families, who remain the major provider of long-term care for the elderly, and the emphasis of current governmental programs.

In the second section of the book, "In-Home Service Programs for the Chronically Limited Elderly: An Analysis of National Policy," we take a closer look at the core service area of community-based long-term care. We begin with a discussion of methodological issues in Chapter 4. Here, we consider the value base underlying our analysis. We discuss the concept of "adequacy," and urge the development of more refined measurements than are currently available. We go on to discuss the concepts of "need" and "disability." The results of several surveys of disability in the elderly are presented, and the problems of converting these estimates into an estimate of need for in-home services are discussed. Also, we discuss the limitations of our assumptions and of the data available to measure currently provided services. This chapter emphasizes the need for more sophisticated, standardized data collection techniques and the need for collection of such data on a systematized national basis. In Chapter 5, we build on the methodological assumptions discussed in Chapter 4. Here, selected aspects of four major in-home service programs which are federally funded are examined. These programs are funded by Medicare, Medicaid, Title XX of the Social Security Act, and Title III of the Older Americans Act. We begin with a state-by-state analysis of service levels for each program. We find that these programs failed to serve the chronically ill elderly on an equitable state-by-state basis. Major inequities between service levels in the various states were apparent in all programs, although they were less severe in the federal Medicare program. We go on to estimate the adequacy of the combined service provided by the four programs—again on a state-by-state basis. Our results demonstrate that the large majority of chronically ill elderly live in states which provide inadequate levels of in-home services. Only a few, primarily Northeastern states, provide "adequate" service according to our operative definitions. We conclude that the system of linkages between federal, state, and local authorities within Medicaid, Title XX and Title III programs, as well as the emphasis on vendor payment arrangements connecting the public sector with private entrepreneurial or voluntary vendors in Medicare, has resulted in a national system of in-home services characterized by significant equity and adequacy problems as well as by lack of clearly established national goals and priorities. We urge that such goals and priorities be articulated at the federal level and be backed by adequate funding and regulatory policy as well as national administrative coordination.

The next section of the book, titled "In-Home Services and the Community-Based Network of Services: The Status of Current Programs and a Review and Critique of Legislative Proposals,'' contains two chapters. In-home services cannot keep the elderly in the community without a wide range of related social and health programs. Chapter 6 includes a discussion of some of the recent demonstration programs which seek to coordinate community-based services, as well as a discussion of some of the critical components of the community-based long-term care package in addition to home health and in-home social care services such as day care, respite care, nutrition, housing programs, and adult foster care. Where data are available, this chapter seeks to determine the extent of service availability of such programs.

In Chapter 7, we describe and critically analyze some recent proposals for national legislation, and recent legislative enactments seeking to improve in-home social services or in-home health services (as well as related community care services) for the chronically limited elderly. Also discussed in this chapter is the potential impact of recent Congressional ''cutbacks'' on the development of in-home services and other community-based services for the chronically ill elderly. Section IV, ''International Policy Considerations Regarding In-Home Services for the Elderly,'' consists of one chapter which provides a brief consideration of how in-home services for the elderly have been organized within some national contexts which emphasize community-based long-term care for the frail elderly.

Having outlined the thrust of our book, we will proceed in this chapter to present a brief survey of the nature of the medical, health, and social service needs of the elderly and their need for expanded in-home and related community-based services. Finally, we will indicate some implications of our study with respect to the development of a national policy emphasizing in-home and other community-based long-term care services for the chronically limited elderly.

Aging and Impairment: The Problem

The aging population in America is increasing rapidly. At the beginning of 1981, over 25 million older Americans made up over 11 percent of the population—''every 9th American.'' As of mid-1980, over 62 percent of older Americans were 65-75 years of age. Over 2.2 million Americans were 85 years of age or older.

A projection of population growth between 1977 and 2035 has indicated that the population of the United States is expected to grow by 40 percent, from 217 million persons to a figure of 304 million. During this period, the population over 65 years of age is expected to more than double. The segments of the elderly population that are expected to grow most rapidly are those between 75 and 84 years of age and those over 85 years of age (U.S. Department of Health, Education, and Welfare, 1978: 17). Elderly individuals are subject to a greater frequency of both acute and chronic illnesses: the more elderly an individual, the greater the possibility of severe chronic limitation. They are particularly subject to such disabilities as arthritis, hearing and visual impairments, hypertension, and heart disease (U.S. Congress, Senate, 1980: XIII-XXV).

The Prospect of Community-Based Care

A number of studies indicate that the elderly prefer, if possible, not to be institutionalized with the onset of chronic disabilities (Bell, 1973; Sussman, 1979). Also, studies have noted rapid functional deterioration of an institutionalized elderly population (Kahana and Coe, 1969; Lieberman, 1967). In contrast, homemaker services and day care centers have helped maintain the functioning of the elderly—in terms of level of contentment, mental functioning, and social activity (Weissert, Wan, and Livieratos, 1980).

We often have been too reliant on institutional nursing home care in situations where a number of chronic disabilities could be dealt with more appropriately and more humanely by community-based care. Such care, inclusive of home health services, homemaker-home health aid services, adult day services, respite care services, and foster care programs as well as other support services, would permit the chronically limited elderly to maintain maximum independence and minimum disruption of life-style.

While the need for community-based care grows, recent changes in the structure of the family have made it more difficult for the family to assure care or support to the chronically limited elderly. Currently about 50 percent of wives work. In addition to the fact that conjugal families often involve two working parents, divorce is an increasingly common phenomenon. Of marriages consummated in 1980, 40 percent will result in divorce. Another trend is an increase in out-of-wedlock births—often by teenage girls. Also, the size of families has declined. Thus, such events as the development of new family forms, an increase in divorce rates, the decline in household size, and a growth of single parent families hinders the ability of the nuclear family to provide care for dependent, often chronically limited, elderly relatives.

The development of a focus on community care has profound implications for the family members of the chronically limited elderly person. Often family caregivers of the aged are old and possibly functionally limited themselves. When the caregiver is a child, it is almost always a daughter or a daughter-in-law. This person has been called the "woman in the middle" (Brody, 1981) or the "sandwich" generation (Miller, 1981). Because of the changes in family structure mentioned, the caregiver is increasingly likely to be divorced or a single parent who is working. Family caregivers often provide many hours of care each day to elderly relatives who are disabled. Clearly this places an enormous strain on the caregiver who is caught between the demands of her parents, her children, her job, and her husband. Thus, in addition to the increased provision of community home care services, it is critical that services be designed with an understanding of the needs of family members (especially caregivers).

What Should Be Done?

It is perhaps in order at this point to reiterate and elaborate on our initial introduction. We believe our study will demonstrate the need for a national program structure for home health and other in-home services for the chronically ill elderly. It also will indicate a need for national support of other community-based services. Clear national goals regarding levels of provision of community-based services must be related to ratios of chronically limited elderly. Indeed, such ratios also would relate to *levels* of disability of such individuals, as in-home social care and home health care are probably not the most beneficial mechanisms of delivery of care to *all* of the disabled elderly. Also, federal funds would be needed for setting up home health and social care agencies in underserved areas, as well as for development of adult day care, foster care, and respite care services. Thus, our study will demonstrate that in order to assure equity of program delivery and to attempt to achieve the goal of adequacy of provision, a program of home health and in-home social care, as well as supportive community-based services, should be developed which would be nationally funded and based on national implementation of national standards. Such programs should emphasize a "family policy" perspective.

REFERENCES

Bell, William B. "Community Care for the Elderly: Alternatives to Institutionalization." *The Gerontologist,* 13 (Fall 1973), 249-354.

Brody, Elaine M. "Women in the Middle and Family Help to Older People." *The Gerontologist,* 21 (October 1981), 471-480.

Kahana, Eva and Coe, Rodney M. "Self and Self-Conceptions of Institutionalized Aged." *The Gerontologist,* 9 (Winter 1969), 264-267.

Lieberman, Morton A. "Institutionalization of the Aged: Effects on Behavior." *Journal of Gerontology,* 24 (July 1969), 338-339.

Miller, Dorothy. "The Sandwich Generation: Adult Children of the Aging." *Social Work,* 26 (September 1981), 419-423.

Sussman, Marvin B. *Social and Economic Supports and Family Environments for the Elderly.* Final Report No. A-316103, Washington, D.C.: Administration on Aging, January, 1979.

U.S. Congress, Senate, Select Committee on Aging. *Developments in Aging: 1980,* Part 1, Report to the Select Committee on Aging, 97th Cong., 1st Sess., March 5, 1980.

U.S. Department of Health, Education, and Welfare, Federal Council on Aging. *Public Policy and the Frail Elderly.* Washington, D.C., December, 1978.

Weissert, William G.; Wan, Thomas T.H.; and Livieratos, Barbara. "Effects and Cost of Day Care and Homemaker Services for the Chronically-Ill: A Randomized Experiment." Washington, D.C.: National Center for Health Services Research, February, 1980.

Chapter 2

The Aged, Their Health and Social Status, and the Family

The profound changes in demography and social values in the United States in the last decades have had and will continue to have important effects on the nature of the American family and on the place of the elderly in the family unit. The major trends affecting the American family today include declining birth and death rates, a shorter childbearing period, high rates of marriage and divorce, increasing rates of women in the labor force, earlier age at retirement, and decline in multigenerational households (Glick, 1979). Prior to considering the relevance of family policy in developing a national system of in-home and community-based services for the care of the chronically limited elderly, a review of the nature of the contemporary American family and the role of the elderly as family members is in order.

Demography

Since 1900, life expectancy at birth has increased 25 years. Today a person can expect to live to about 74 years (U.S. Bureau of the Census, 1981: 69). This increased longevity (along with declining birth rates) has resulted in a larger and larger proportion of the U.S. population who are over 65 years of age. In 1981, one out of nine Americans was over 65. This compares to one out of fifty in 1776 and one out of 25 in 1900 (U.S. Congress, Senate, 1980). Estimates of the elderly in the population for the year 2000 range from a low of 11.9 percent of the total population to a high of 16 percent depending upon different assumptions regarding birth rate and longevity. Another way to look at this increase is to consider the changing ratio of persons 18-64 to those 65 and over. In 1930 there were 9.1 persons 65+ for every 100 persons 18-64 years of age. By 1980, there were 18.4 persons 65+ for every 100 18-64 year olds.

By the year 2020, there are projected to be 26 older persons for every 100 younger adults (U.S. Congress, Senate, 1980).

Geographically, the state with the highest proportion of persons 65 and over is Florida. The next highest concentrations of elderly persons are in Arkansas, Rhode Island, Iowa, Missouri, South Dakota, Nebraska, Pennsylvania, and Massachusetts (see Table 1 and Figure 1).

Of the two groups of elderly, the young-old and the old-old, it is well known that it is the oldest group which is growing at the fastest rate. For example, between 1976 and 2000, the population 65-74 is expected to increase 22.8 percent; those 75-84 will increase by 56.9 percent and those 85 and over will increase 91.1 percent. Females over 84 are expected to increase by over 100 percent (U.S. Congress, Senate, 1980).

The growth of the older population increases the likelihood of a four generation family. As people are living longer and at the same time marrying and having children younger, the child-bearing period becomes a stage of life rather than an activity which extends through adulthood. The "empty nest" period (from when the last child leaves home) has lengthened. Thus the modern family can be seen going through a series of stages from marriage, child-bearing and rearing, a period when working husband and wife live alone, a period when retired husband and wife live alone to widowhood and death.

Another important consideration is that life expectancy has not increased equally for men and women. Longevity has increased for women at a greater rate than for men. In 1900, life expectancy for women was 48 and for men 46. The discrepancy was about two years. In 1978, life expectation for white males was 70.2 years, while for white females it was 77.8 years. Figures for non-whites were 65 and 73.6 respectively (U.S. Bureau of the Census, 1980: 73). Thus the differential is now about 8 years. Also, as of 1980, about one out of every six elderly persons had an annual income below the poverty level (see Figure 2). This ratio represents a long-term decline in poverty among the elderly due in large part to improvements in social security benefits.

Marital Status

Because of this differential life expectancy of men and women, most older men are married (about 75 percent) and most older women are widows. This tendency becomes more pronounced as

TABLE 1

NUMBER AND PERCENT OF EACH STATE'S TOTAL POPULATION AGED 65 AND OVER,
1980 CENSUS COUNT (APR. 1)

[Numbers in thousands]

State	All ages Number	All ages Rank	65 plus Number	65 plus Rank	65 plus Percent	65 plus Rank	Percent Increase 1970-80
Alabama	3,890	22	440	19	11.3	24	35.8
Alaska	400	51	12	51	2.9	51	71.4
Arizona	2,718	29	307	28	11.3	25	90.7
Arkansas	2,286	33	312	27	13.7	2	31.6
California	23,669	1	2,415	1	10.2	34	34.8
Colorado	2,889	28	247	33	8.6	46	32.1
Connecticut	3,108	25	365	26	11.7	18	26.7
Delaware	595	48	59	48	10.0	36	34.1
District of Columbia	638	47	74	46	11.6	20	5.7
Florida	9,740	7	1,685	3	17.3	1	71.1
Georgia	5,464	13	517	16	9.5	41	41.6
Hawaii	965	39	76	45	7.9	49	72.7
Idaho	944	41	94	41	9.9	37	40.3
Illinois	11,418	5	1,261	6	11.0	29	15.8
Indiana	5,490	12	585	13	10.7	31	18.9
Iowa	2,913	27	387	24	13.3	4	10.9
Kansas	2,363	32	306	29	13.0	8	15.5
Kentucky	3,661	23	410	21	11.2	27	22.0
Louisiana	4,204	19	404	22	9.6	39	32.5
Maine	1,125	38	141	36	12.5	11	23.7
Maryland	4,216	18	396	23	9.4	42	32.9
Massachusetts	5,737	11	727	10	12.7	10	14.8
Michigan	9,258	8	912	8	9.8	38	21.8
Minnesota	4,077	21	480	18	11.8	17	17.9
Mississippi	2,521	31	289	31	11.5	21	30.8
Missouri	4,917	15	648	11	13.2	5	16.1
Montana	787	44	85	43	10.7	32	25.0
Nebraska	1,570	35	206	35	13.1	7	12.6
Nevada	799	43	66	47	8.2	47	113.0
New Hampshire	921	42	103	40	11.2	28	32.1
New Jersey	7,364	9	860	9	11.7	19	23.9
New Mexico	1,300	37	116	38	8.9	45	65.7
New York	17,557	2	2,161	2	12.3	13	10.8
North Carolina	5,874	10	602	12	10.2	35	46.1
North Dakota	653	46	80	44	12.3	14	21.2
Ohio	10,797	6	1,169	7	10.8	30	17.7
Oklahoma	3,025	26	376	25	12.4	12	25.8
Oregon	2,633	30	303	30	11.5	22	34.1
Pennsylvania	11,867	4	1,531	4	12.9	9	20.8
Phode Island	947	40	127	37	13.4	3	22.1
South Carolina	3,119	24	287	32	9.2	44	51.1
South Dakota	690	45	91	42	13.2	6	13.8
Tennessee	4,591	17	518	15	11.3	26	35.6
Texas	14,228	3	1,371	5	9.6	40	38.8
Utah	1,461	36	109	39	7.5	50	41.4
Vermont	511	49	58	49	11.4	23	23.4
Virginia	5,346	14	505	17	9.4	43	38.7
Washington	4,130	20	431	20	10.4	33	31.7
West Virginia	1,950	34	238	34	12.2	15	22.7
Wisconsin	4,705	16	564	14	12.0	16	19.7
Wyoming	471	50	38	50	8.0	48	66.7

Source: U.S. Congress, Senate, Special Committee on Aging, *Developments in Aging: 1981*, Vol. 1, Report, 97th Cong., 2nd Sess., 1982, p. 30.

FIGURE 1.

PERCENT OF STATE POPULATION AGED 65 AND OVER
1980

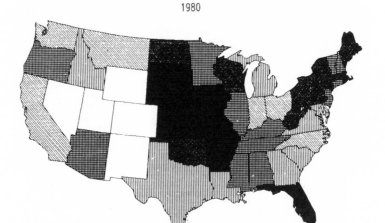

SOURCE: 1980 CENSUS DATA

PERCENT INCREASE IN STATE POPULATION AGED 65 AND OVER

1970 – 1980

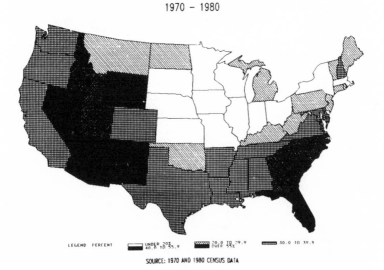

SOURCE: 1970 AND 1980 CENSUS DATA

Cited in U.S. Congress, Senate. *Developments in Aging: 1981*, Vol. 1, Report of the Special Committee on Aging, 97th Cong., 2nd Sess., 1982, p. 31.

FIGURE 2. Percent of Older and Total Population with Income below the Official Poverty Level, Selected Years 1959-1980.

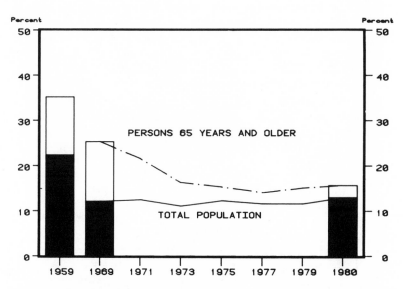

Source: U.S. Current Population Report, Series P-60, No. 127. Cited in U.S. Congress, Senate. *Developments in Aging: 1981*, Vol. 1, Report of the Special Committee on Aging, 97th Cong., 2nd Sess., 1982, p. 24.

age increases, thus while 40 percent of women 65-74 are widowed, 68 percent of those 75 and over are widows (United States Bureau of the Census, 1978). There are 100 women to every 69 men in the 65 and over category. For this reason, as well as the tendency of men to marry younger women, widowed men remarry at a rate of 8 times higher than widowed women (Brotman, 1980).

Living Arrangements

The most common living arrangement for people over 65 is the two-member family: husband and wife living alone. Because there are so many more widows than widowers, more elderly men live with their spouses (75 percent) than do women (33 percent). As age increases, the chance of living alone or in an institutional setting increases for both sexes. In 1980, almost 40 percent of all women

over age 65 lived alone. This compared with a rate of 15 percent for
all men over 65 (U.S. Congress, Senate, 1982: 14). The living arrangements of mature and older women are illustrated in Figure 3.
However, the family remains the most common type of living arrangement, even for those over 75. Seventy-five percent of men and
49 percent of women over 75 live in a family setting. Older women
living with families are more likely than are older men to be living
with relatives other than spouses.

It is often assumed that in the past older persons lived in larger,
multigeneration families. Recent analysis (Dahlin, 1980; Mindel,
1979) shows that while the proportion of older persons living with
their children has been decreasing, it was never the prominent pat-

FIGURE 3. Living Arrangements of Mature and Older Women: 1980.

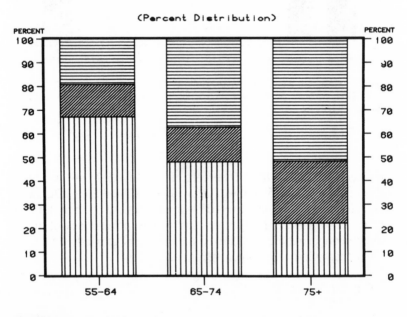

(Percent Distribution)

 WITH SPOUSE
WITH RELATIVE
ALONE OR WITH NON-RELATIVE

Note: Data pertain to
the noninstitutional
population.

Source: U.S. Current Population Report, Series P-20, No. 365. Cited in U.S. Congress,
Senate. *Developments in Aging: 1981,* Vol. 1, Report of the Special Committee on Aging,
97th Cong., 2nd Sess., 1982, p. 15.

tern. In 1940, 15 percent of males and 30 percent of females over 65 were living in households as "other relatives"—neither head nor spouse of head. By 1975, these figures had fallen to 4 percent and 13 percent respectively (Mindel, 1979). Today, most older widows live alone, and only 20 percent live with another family member (National Council on Aging, 1979). The decline in shared households is a result of increased availability of housing following World War II, rising incomes which make separate households possible, and changing live-styles often related to employment responsibilities. If recent reverses in these trends continue, there might be an increase in the multigeneration household in the next few decades.

Health Status

While today's elderly may be more healthy than in the past, there is an increasing likelihood of functional limitation due to illness as age increases (Kovar, 1977). Eighty-five percent of those over 65 have at least one chronic illness, and many have a number of chronic problems at once (U.S., Department of Health, Education, and Welfare, National Center for Health Statistics, 1976). A special study conducted by the U.S. General Accounting Office (GAO) for the Federal Council on Aging showed a relationship between "impairment" and aging[1] (see Table 2). The study noted an almost doubling of the "extremely impaired" rate between the 75-79 age group and the 80-84 age group.

While older persons made up 11 percent of the population in 1978, they accounted for 29.4 percent of the personal health care costs. As would be expected given the distribution of illness in the population, utilization of health care facilities is highest in the oldest sectors of the population (Table 3). Thus the oldest population is not only likely to be female and widowed, but beset with chronic health problems which bring about heavy utilization of health care facilities.

Two Groups of Elderly

In considering the family life of the elderly, there are two stages and sets of relationships which may be involved. A couple in their sixties or early seventies may be relatively healthy. They may have

---

[1]See note following Table 2.

Table 2

DETAILED BREAK-DOWN OF WELL-BEING STATUS BY AGE

	Percent of Age Group				
Well-Being Status *	Under 70	70-74	75-79	80-84	85+
Unimpaired	25.8	20.5	14.9	8.7	9.2
Slightly Impaired	25.1	25.0	15.7	15.0	11.2
Mildly Impaired	19.2	19.5	21.0	21.4	22.5
Moderately Impaired	13.7	12.1	22.6	17.9	14.3
Generally Impaired	5.4	10.8	9.3	11.6	12.2
Greatly Impaired	1.9	2.9	3.6	2.9	2.0
Very Greatly Impaired	2.6	2.4	3.6	4.6	6.1
Extremely Impaired	6.3	6.8	9.3	17.9	22.5
	100	100	100	100	100

Source: U.S. Department of Health, Education, and Welfare, Federal Council on
         Aging. Public Policy and the Frail Elderly, Washington, D.C., December,
         1978, p. 29.

*Note to Table 2

The categories of well-being in this figure come from the Older Americans
Rating Scale developed by the Duke University Center for the Study of Aging
and Human Development and the Administration on Aging. Questions were asked
to older persons in five areas of functioning: 1. social, 2. economic,
3. mental, 4. physical, and 5. activities of daily living. In each of the five
areas, each respondent was scored in one of six categories: excellent, good,
mildly impaired, moderately impaired, severely impaired, or totally impaired.
For example, physical health was rated as follows:

1. In excellent physical health.
    Engages in vigorous physical activity, either
    regularly or at least from time to time.

2. In good physical health.
    No significant illnesses or disabilities. Only
    routine medical care such as annual checkups required.

3. Mildly physically impaired.
    Has only minor illnesses and/or disabilities which might
    benefit from medical treatment or corrective measures.

4. Moderately physically impaired.
    Has one or more diseases or disabilities which are
    either painful or require substantial medical treatment.

5. Severely physically impaired.
    Has one or more illnesses or disabilities which are
    either severely painful or life threatening or
    require extensive medical treatment.

6. Totally physically impaired.
    Confined to bed and requiring full-time medical
    assistance or nursing care to maintain vital
    bodily functions.

Table 2 (continued)

In order to develop an overall score for the functioning, or well-being of
each respondent, scores in the five areas were combined into a total score as
follows:

Impairment level	Description based on five areas included in Duke University questionnaire
Unimpaired	Excellent or good in all five areas of human functioning.
Slightly impaired	Excellent or good in four areas.
Mildly impaired	Mildly or moderately impaired in two areas or mildly or moderately impaired in one area and severely or completely impaired in another.
Moderately impaired	Mildly or moderately impaired in three areas and or mildly or moderately impaired in two and severely or completely impaired in one.
Generally impaired	Mildly or moderately impaired in four areas.
Greatly impaired	Mildly or moderately impaired in three areas, and severely or completely impaired in another.
Very greatly impaired	Mildly or moderately impaired in all five areas.
Extremely impaired	Mildly or moderately impaired in four areas and severely or completely impaired in the other, or severely or completely impaired in two or more areas.

Table 3

Utilization of Hospital and Nursing Home Facilities

Age Group	Average Length of Stay	
	Hospital	Nursing Home
55-64	1.9 days	1 day
65-74	3.2 days	4.4 days
75-84		21.5 days
	6.0 days	
85+		86.4 days

Source: U.S. Congress, Senate, Special Committee on Aging. *Developments in Aging: 1981*,
Part 1, Report, 97th Cong., 1st Sess., 1981, p. xxv.

family interaction with their children and grandchildren as well as siblings. They may also interact with their own parents (or parent) who would be in their eighties or nineties. The family life of a person in his/her eighties would be quite different. These persons are most probably widows who live alone or with their children. They may have interaction with children, grandchildren, and great-grandchildren as well as (possibly) siblings. The distinction here is between the young-old and the old-old. It is the old-old group which is the most likely to be ill or disabled. The type of interaction and of exchange in these two types of elderly families would be quite different. In discussing the family life of the elderly, it is important to distinguish between these two types. As our concern in this chapter is with the impaired elderly, we are likely to find the impaired elderly in the old-old group, while the family caregiver will most likely be part of the young-old group (Gelfand, Olsen, and Block, 1978; Brody, 1980; Miller, 1981).

In the remainder of this chapter, we will discuss the family life of the elderly, assess the family support available to the impaired elderly now, and discuss prospects for the future.

Family Support of the Aged

The fact that most elderly do not live with their relatives (other than spouses) does not mean that they are isolated from them. While classical sociology has argued that we are evolving an isolated nuclear family, recent evidence supports the view that we have a modified extended family system which maintains ties and supports over geographic distance (Litwak, 1959; Sussman, 1955; Dobrof and Litwak, 1977). While only about 10 percent of elderly persons currently live with their children, a number of studies (Townsend, 1957; Shanas et al., 1968; Mahoney, 1977) have documented the fact that a high percentage of elderly parents live close to at least one child. About 75 percent of elderly parents live within a half hour drive of at least one child; moreover, a study by Mahoney (based on 1974 data) indicated that 80 percent of the elderly respondents had face-to-face contact with their children within the previous two weeks.

In considering help exchanges between the elderly and their families, the distinction between the young-old and the old-old is especially important. The young-old family is likely to be a relatively healthy couple living alone. While we tend to think of the elderly as recipients of help from their families, in fact, aid is exchanged in both directions (Streib, 1958; Riley and Forner, 1968; and Sussman, 1953). The young-old often provide housing, financial aid, emotional support, child care, housework, and companionship to their children and grandchildren.

The major problem which requires the elderly to turn to family members for help is illness. Families now provide 80 percent of the home health care services for older relatives (NCHS, 1972), and a substantial proportion of the long-term care in the United States is provided by family members (U.S. Congressional Budget Office, 1977). A study by Cantor and Johnson of 1,552 New York City elderly found that of 224 respondents who were sick a week or less, 60 percent received care from family members, and 12 percent from friends and neighbors; 4 percent received care through formal organizations, while 28 percent received no help at all. For those who suffered an illness of between one and two weeks duration, 70 percent reported that they received care from family members; 15 percent indicated that they received care from friends and neighbors; 3 percent received care from formal organizations, and 16 percent received no care from anyone.

Widespread acceptance of familial responsibility for the elderly exists; according to Sussman (1977), 81 percent of families have indicated that they would agree to take in an older relative under some circumstances. In fact, the probability of an elderly person living with adult children is negatively related to his or her level of health.

While the institutionalized elderly are often depicted as having been abandoned by their families, in fact many of them are widows without children or never-married men or women. Those institutionalized elderly with families have often exhausted the financial and psychological resources of the family, and were institutionalized as a last resort (Eggert and Granger, 1977; Brody, 1978). A significant question is whether a professional service delivery structure of community-based care would have prevented some of such institutionalization.

Several factors appear to be related to help patterns in American families. Mahoney (1977) found that the rural and suburban elderly are more likely to receive needed help from family members than urban and small town situated elderly. Also, Moroney (1976) determined that lower income groups are more likely to provide physical and household help to the chronically limited elderly, while middle income groups were more likely to help out financially. Social-economic status (SES) also appears to be related to intrafamilial relationships. In middle-class families, ties are strongest between females. In lower-class families, ties follow a same sex pattern, with men close to men, and women to women. Patterns of residential proximity also vary according to class. While lower-class families may reside in close proximity throughout the life cycle, the middle-class family may go through a period after children gain independence where distances between residences are great. However, there is some evidence that children move closer to their parents as the parents age. (Troll et al., 1979). Even in families who do not live near each other, frequent interaction is maintained through telephone and mail contact.

American families have diverse cultural and ethnic heritages. It is often thought that ethnic families are stronger and more cohesive than the typical white Anglo-Saxon American family. Thus we might expect even more interaction and mutual aid in these families. There is evidence that this is true in Hispanic (Maldonado, 1979) and Oriental (Weeks and Cuellar, 1981) families. However, there is no evidence that there is more help exchanged in Black families (Cantor, 1979). One explanation is that when people arrive in the United States as immigrants, family values are strong. However, over time, the success orientation of American culture gains more importance, and the family takes a position congruent with that in American culture (Gelfand and Fandetti, 1980). Recent immigration to the United States from countries such as Taiwan, the Philippines, Japan, India, Korea, Vietnam, Mexico, Cuba, Greece, and Italy might indicate a strong family orientation within these ethnic groups for some time to come.

Caregiving by the Spouse

When illness occurs in the young-old family, help is usually provided by the spouse. Given the differential in life expectancy between men and women, the fact that women marry older men, and the relationship between age and functional limitations, the most common pattern will be for the wife to be the caregiver for her ailing husband. When husbands become ill, wives are likely to take on nursing functions. This can be as minimal as watching diet and encouraging exercise to what amounts to full-time nursing care for a bedridden spouse. This situation can be expected to alter the marital relationship, with the husband needing to adjust to a dependent role and the wife to taking on a heavy caretaking burden as well as increased responsibility. In a traditional marriage, these adjustments may be very difficult. When an extensive period of caregiving precedes the death of the spouse, caregiving responsibilities may serve to cut the caregiving spouse off from friends and social activities, and this may make the adjustment to widowhood even more difficult. Research on the impact of caring for an ill spouse is relatively recent; however, preliminary results show that emotional strain is common, and that this strain is felt primarily by the spouse. Things most likely to be sacrificed by the caregiver are free time, social activities, running errands, and vacations (Cantor, 1980). Prolonged strain of this type could be expected to have negative effects on the caregiver's physical and mental health.

Caregiving by the Children

It is clear that the large majority of American elderly have a strong preference for independent living. They also try to adhere to the norm that the aged should not make demands on adult children. They seem to be concerned that imposing too much will lead to resentment and, ultimately, rejection. Thus too little contact is seen to be better (or safer) than too much. There is also evidence that relationships with adult children are not highly rewarding to the elderly, nor do they boost morale as do relationships with friends. While contact may be frequent and expressed satisfaction with the relationship may be high, the relations between the elderly and their adult children may not be intimate. Instead, conversation may be a type of catching up or checking up, with get-togethers made up of rituals around holidays and family occasions (Lowenthal and Robinson, 1976). In spite of the desire for independent functioning, an older person who becomes ill or disabled and does not have a spouse is most likely to seek help from his/her children.

There is some evidence of a sexual division of labor among offsprings in the provision of help for elderly parents. Sons are more likely to provide financial help, while it is daughters who take parents in, visit, and provide emotional support for personal care (Lopata, 1973; Simos, 1973). Even when sons take ill mothers in, it is usually the daughter-in-law who actually provides the care. Another important factor is the number of siblings available to share the caregiving responsibilities (Johnson and Bursk, 1977; Simos, 1973).

Blau (1973) suggests that sickness demoralizes elderly people and alienates those close to them. When a parent becomes ill, a role-reversal occurs in which the child becomes the caregiver and the elderly parent becomes dependent. This can cause resentment, anger, and depression on the part of the elderly parent, who mourns for the loss of health and independence. It can also cause resentment in the child, who mourns for the loss of his parent and of his freedom. The serious illness of an elderly parent creates a crisis for the child because he recognizes the mortality of the parent. This will make the child the next oldest generation. The fact that many of the old-old suffer from mental as well as physical deterioration is additionally stressful to children. The decision surrounding the institutionalization of a parent can raise previously buried family conflicts and create a crisis for the entire family (Cath, 1970). Such conflicts often are reborn when an aged parent comes to live with a child. Long buried feelings of rejection and sibling rivalry can reemerge (Savitsky and Sharkey, 1972).

In sum, aged persons in good health can expect to keep in close touch with their children. They are likely to continue to provide help to children, and to maintain an important, although not necessarily an active, role in their children's lives. When physical or mental health deteriorates, however, strains in the relationship may occur. This is especially true if the elderly person moves in with the adult child and requires extensive care.

Other Caregiving Patterns   "hierarchy of responsibility"

The determination of a "caregiver" seems to follow a hierarchical pattern. First preference is the spouse. If there is no spouse, or he/she is incapable of providing care, then children are "caregivers of choice." If there are no children, or if children are unable or unwilling to help, the elderly will seek out help from other relatives in preference to aid from community or governmental agencies (Shanas et al., 1968). This "hierarchy of responsibility" was identified by Cantor (1980). The impact of caregiving on relatives other than spouse or children has not been studied. There is some evidence that this type of pattern (caregiving by other relatives) may be more common in Black families than in other American families.

A number of observers, then, have suggested that caring for elderly sick relatives is stressful and may even result in the physical and/or mental breakdown of caregivers (Newman, 1976; Sanford, 1975; Eggert et al., 1977; Krumpoltz, in progress). There is some evidence that the strain is greater when the caregiver is a child (daughter) than when the spouse (wife) provides care. In this case, satisfaction with care is also lower (Lurie, 1981).

The Future of Family Caregiving

Given the importance of the support provided to the elderly by the family—especially in the area of health care, the ability of the family to continue to provide this care is critical. What factors will affect the family caregiving function in the future?

One demographic change which will have profound implications for the ability of the family to provide support for the aged in the future is the declining birth rate. While today's elderly person is likely to have been born into a family of five children, he is likely to have had about three, and his children have only one or two children. In 1980 family size averaged 3.27 persons (U.S. Department of Commerce, 1981b). The declining birth rate means that there will be fewer adult children available to support aged parents in the future. As care of the elderly is traditionally provided by the female child, it is possible to calculate the number of women available for support. Kobrin (1976) estimated that while in 1910 there were 3 women aged 35-44 for every widow and divorcee aged 55 and older, by 1973 there were only 1.2. Thus the number of potential caregivers has declined substantially and can be expected to decline even further in the future. In addition, marriage rates have eliminated the "maiden aunts" who in the past had often been most available for care of the elderly.

Another important change has come in the area of women's roles. Married women are far more likely to work outside of the home than was the case earlier in the century. For example, in 1940, 11 percent of married women aged 45-54 were working compared with 51 percent in 1977 (U.S. Bureau of the Census, 1973; Young, U.S. Bureau of Labor Statistics, 1979: A21). The average number of working wives rose from 32 percent in 1947 to almost 51 percent in 1978 (Hayghe, 1981: 47). In 1977, the traditional style of family with the husband in the workforce and the wife and children at home accounted for only 15 percent of American families. An increasing proportion of husband-wife families have wives in the labor force (B. Johnson, 1978: 33), while an increasing percentage of families are headed by a single male or female parent (Hayghe, 1976; U.S. Department of Commerce, 1981a: 3). The tendency for women to work can be expected to be strengthened if the recent trends of slower entry into marriage, high divorce rates, and inflation persist. It is unclear how the fact that more women are working will effect the family's ability to help elderly relatives. If these women retire at 60 or 65, they are likely to be retired or close to retirement at the time when they might be called upon to help an elderly relative. However, it is clear that the trend is toward later retirement. Thus it is increasingly likely that the elderly widow who becomes ill will be dependent upon a working daughter. In addition, if the tendency for women to postpone childbearing until the mid or late thirties continues, this daughter is also likely to be carrying considerable responsibility toward her young adult children.

Finally, the dramatic rise in divorce rates since 1970 can be expected to affect the ability of families to care for impaired elderly relatives. As we have noted earlier, today about 40 percent of recent marriages can be expected to end in divorce (Uhlenberg and Myers, 1981). Although the highest rates of divorce occur in the younger cohorts (25-39 years), divorce rates have doubled in older cohorts as well. In 1978, there were about 100 divorced women for every 1,000 women, or 1 in 10. For men, the number divorced has risen, but not so dramatically. There were about 60 divorced men per 1,000 in this age group in 1978. This is because men are more likely to remarry (U.S. Department of Commerce, 1980). And because so many divorced persons later remarry, the number who have been divorced among both the young-old and the old-old populations is actually more like 25 percent. In the future, these numbers can be expected to be much higher.

How will these divorce rates affect the impaired elderly? Obviously, if not remarried, the divorced will not have the spouse to provide care in case of illness or disability. Secondly, divorced women in the young-old generation will be more likely to work and thus may be less available to older relatives. Finally, it is possible that divorces in earlier days may create strain in parent-child relationships which could effect the willingness of the child to provide caregiving to the parent when he or she is old.

For these reasons (low birth rates, women working, and high divorce rates), we must look upon the family as a declining source of support for the elderly. This in no way suggests that people are unwilling to provide assistance to elderly relatives. Rather, there will be fewer related persons in the appropriate age brackets per elderly person, and these may have competition for their limited resources from work, children, and grandchildren. As Callahan et al. (1980) have noted:

> The proliferation of new family forms, coupled with an increase in divorce, decline in household size, and growth in single parent families, raises the question of whether the nuclear family can even give personal care to those members who need it. One outcome of an increased participation in the labor force has been to raise the price of family members caring for the homebound. Potential income foregone is a real opportunity cost becoming more visible to those who must remain at home.

Conclusion

In planning future policy, it is important to recognize differences between cohorts of elderly. We cannot set policy for the year 2000 based on our knowledge of those who are elderly today. In fact, many of the trends we have been discussing are recent and would not be expected to affect the elderly directly for several decades.

Those who are now old were often immigrants from other countries or migrants from rural to urban areas. They are likely to hold "traditional" values of family responsibility, and to want to be independent of extra-familial assistance. On the other hand, persons who become elderly after the turn of the century (the baby-boom generation) have been most profoundly affected by the trends we have discussed in this section. They have smaller families, larger numbers have no children, the divorce rate has been very high in this cohort, and single parent, stepparent, and alternative families are not uncommon. Also, profound changes in the traditional woman's role have occurred in this cohort, with women achieving higher educational and occupational status than ever before. This generation has also been active in political and human rights movements. This experience may make them a sophisticated and politically powerful group of aged.

In sum, the family is a major resource for the elderly person who becomes ill. For the young-old, the caregiver is often the spouse. For the old-old it is more likely to be a child, especially a daughter. In fact, as the elderly person in need of care from a child is likely to be very old, the "child" providing care is often old herself. In the four-generation family, it is the young-old generation—the retired couple who are providing care for the old-old generation.

Nevertheless, there are indications that the family will not be able to continue the current high degree of care of the elderly without financial and service supports. The changing age structure and life expectancy of the population are increasing the number of vulnerable elderly persons who are in need of long-term care. At the same time, declining birth rates, high divorce rates, and high proportions of women in the labor force may be reducing the ability of the family to provide care.

In our next chapter, we will consider the family policy concept as a guide for the development of community-based health and social services for the elderly and their families.

REFERENCES

Albrecht, Ruth. "The Parental Responsibilities of Grandparents." *Marriage and Family Living*, 16 (August 1954), 201-204.
Atchley, Robert C. "Dimensions of Widowhood in Later Life." *The Gerontologist*, 15 (April 1975), 176-178.
Atchley, Robert C. *Social Forces in Later Life*. Belmont, California: Wadsworth, 1972.
Blenkner, Margaret. "Social Work and Family Relationships in Later Life With Some Thoughts on Filial Maturity," in Ethel Shanas and Gordon Streib (eds.), *Social Structure and The Family*. Englewood Cliffs, N.J.: Prentice-Hall, 1965, pp. 46-59.
Blau, Zena S. *Old Age in a Changing Society*. New York: New Viewpoints, a division of Franklin Watts, Inc., 1973.
Block, Marilyn R.; Davidson, J. L.; Grants, J. D.; and Serock, K. E. *Uncharted Territories, Issues and Concerns of Women Over 40*. College Park, Maryland: University of Maryland, Center on Aging, 1978.
Block, Marilyn R. and Simmott, J. D. (eds.). *The Battered Elder Syndrome: An Exploratory Study*. College Park, Maryland: University of Maryland, Center on Aging, 1979.
Bloom, Martin and Monroe, A. "Social Work and the Aging Family." *The Family Coordinator* (January 1972), 103-113.
Brickner, Philip W. *Home Health Care for the Aged: How to Help Older People Stay in Their Own Homes and Out of Institutions*. New York: Appleton-Century-Crofts, 1978.
Brody, Elaine M. "The Aging of the Family." *The Annals, ASPSS*, 430 (July 1978), 13-27.
Brody, Elaine M. "The Aging Family." *The Gerontologist*, 6 (December 1966), 201-206.
Brody, Elaine M. and Brody, Stanley J. "Decade of Decision for the Elderly." *Social Work*, 19 (September 1974), 544-554.
Brotman, Herman. "Every Ninth American," in *Developments in Aging*. U.S. Senate, Special Committee on Aging, 1980.
Brown, Robert G. "Family Structure and Social Isolation of Older Persons." *Journal of Gerontology*, 15 (April 1960), 170-173.
Butler, Robert N. *Why Survive? Being Old in America*. New York: Harper and Row, 1975.
Cantor, Marjorie H. "Life Space and the Social Support System of the Inner-City Elderly of New York." *Gerontologist*, 15 (February 1975), 23-26.

Howard A. Palley and Julianne S. Oktay   29

Cantor, Marjorie H. "Caring for the Frail Elderly: Impact on Family, Friends and Neighbors." Presented at Gerontological Society Meeting, San Diego, 1980.

Cath, Stanley H. "The Geriatric Patient and His Family—The Institutionalization of a Parent—A Nadir of Life." Gerontology Society Presentation, 1970.

Christopherson, V. A. "Family Reactions to Illness,'" in *Living in the Multigeneration Family.* Ann Arbor: The University of Michigan, 1969.

Clavan, Sylvia. "The Impact of Social Class and Social Trends on the Role of Grandparent." *The Family Coordinator,* 27 (October 1978), 351-357.

Cleveland, William P. and Gianturco, Daniel T. "Remarriage Probability After Widowhood: A Retrospective Method." *Journal of Gerontology,* 31 (January 1976), 99-103.

Cohn, Stephen Z. and Gans, B. M. *The Other Generation Gap: The Middle-Aged and Their Aging Parents.* Chicago: Follett Pub. Corp., 1978.

Coward, R. T. "Planning Community Services for the Rural Elderly: Implications from Research." *The Gerontologist,* 19 (June 1979), 275-282.

Dahlin, Michel. "Perspectives on the Family Life of the Elderly in 1900." *The Gerontologist,* 20 (February 1980), 99-107.

Davidson, J. L. "Elder Abuse," in M. R. Block and J. D. Simmott (eds.), *The Battered Elder Syndrome: An Exploratory Study.* College Park, Maryland: University of Maryland, Center on Aging, 1979, pp. 49-55.

deBeauvoir, Simone, *The Coming of Age.* New York: G. P. Putnam's Sons, 1972.

Dobrof, Rose and Litwak, Eugene. *Maintenance of Family Ties of Long-Term Care Patients: Theory and Guide to Practice.* Washington, D.C.: U.S. Government Printing Office, 1977.

Donahue, W. "Living in the Four-Generation Family," in *Living in the Multigeneration Family.* Ann Arbor: The University of Michigan, 1969.

Eggert, Gerald; Granger, M. C. et al. "Caring for the Patient With Long-Term Disability," *Journal of the American Geriatric Society* (October 1977), 102-114.

Fandetti, Donald and Gelfand, Donald. "Caring of the Aged: Attitudes of White Ethnic Families." *Gerontologist,* 16 (December 1976), 544-549.

Fengler, Alfred F. "Attitudinal Orientations of Wives Toward Their Husband's Retirement." *International Journal of Aging and Human Development,* 6 (2, 1975), 139-152.

Fischer, D. H. *Growing Old in America.* New York: Oxford University Press, 1977.

Gelfand, Donald; Olsen, Jody; and Block, Marilyn. "The Two Generation Geriatric Family." *The Family Coordinator,* 27 (October 1978), 395-403.

Glick, Paul C. "The Future of the American Family." *Current Population Reports.* Special Studies, Series P-3, No. 78, January 1979.

Goldfarb, Alvin I. "Psychodynamics and the Three-Generation Family," in Ethel Shanas and Gordon Streib (eds.), *Social Structure and the Family: Generational Relations.* Englewood Cliffs, N.J.: Prentice-Hall, 1965, pp. 10-45.

Gubrium, Jaber F. (ed.). *Time, Roles, and Self in Old Age.* New York: Human Science Press, 1976.

Hayghe, Howard. "Husbands and Wives as Earners: An Analysis of Family Data." *Monthly Labor Review,* 104 (February 1981), 46-53.

Hays, W. C. and Mindel, C. H. "Extended Kinship Relations in Black and White Families," in *Marriage and the Family: Generational Relations.* Englewood Cliffs, N.J.: Prentice-Hall, 1965.

Huling, William. "Evolving Family Roles for the Black Elderly." *Aging* (October 1978), 21-27.

Isaacs, Bernard; Livingstone, M.; and Neville, Y. *Survival of the Unfittest.* Boston: Routledge and Kegan Paul, 1972.

Johnson, Elizabeth S. and Bursk, Barbara J. "Relationships Between the Elderly and Their Adult Children." *Gerontologist,* 17 (February 1977), 90-96.

Johnson, Beverly L. "Women Who Head Families, 1970-77, Their Numbers, Race, Income Logged." *Monthly Labor Review,* 101 (February 1978), 32-37.

Kaplan, Jerome. "The Family in Aging." *The Gerontologist,* 15 (October 1975), 385.

30   THE CHRONICALLY LIMITED ELDERLY

Kirschner, Charlotte. "The Aging Family in Crisis." *Social Casework*, 60 (1979), 209-216.
Kobrin, Francis E. "The Fall of Household Size and the Rise of the Primary Individual in the United States." *Demography*, 13 (February 1976), 127-138.
Kovar, Mary Grace. "Health of the Elderly and Use of Health Services." *Public Health Reports*, 92 (January-February 1977), 9-21.
Lebowitz, Barry D. "Old Age and Family Functioning." *Journal of Gerontological Social Work*, 1 (Winter 1978), 111-118.
Litwak, Eugene. "Extended Kin Relations in an Industrial Democratic Society," in Ethel Shanas and Gordon Streib (eds.), *Social Structure and the Family: Generational Relations*. Englewood Cliffs, N.J.: Prentice-Hall, 1965, pp. 290-323.
Lopata, Helen Z. *Widowhood in an American City*. Schenkman, Cambridge, 1973.
Lowenthal, M. F. and Robinson, Betsy. "Social Networks and Isolation," in Robert Binstock and Ethel Shanas (eds.), *Handbook of Aging and the Social Sciences*. New York: Van Nostrand Reinhold, 1976, pp. 432-456.
Lowy, Louis. *Social Work With the Aging: The Challenge and Promise of the Later Years*. New York: Harper and Row, 1979.
Lurie, Elinor. "Formal and Informal Supports in the Post-Hospital Period." Presented at the Gerontological Society of America. Toronto, 1981.
Maldonado, David. "Aging in the Chicano Context," in Donald E. Gelfand and Alfred J. Kutzik (eds.), *Ethnicity and Aging: Theory, Research, and Policy*. New York: Springer Pub., 1979, pp. 175-183.
Maldonado, David. "The Chicano Aged." *Social Work*, 20 (May 1975), 213-216.
Miller, Michael B. "The Chronically Ill Aged, Family Conflict, and Family Medicine." *American Geriatrics Society Journal*, 17 (9, 1969), 950-969.
Miller, Dorothy A. "The 'Sandwich' Generation: Adult Children of the Aging." *Social Work*, 10 (September 1981), 419-423.
Mindel, Charles H. "Multigenerational Family Household: Recent Trends and Implications for the Future." *The Gerontologist*, 19 (October 1979), 456-463.
Monk, Abraham. "Family Supports in Old Age." *Social Work*, 24 (November 1979), 533-538.
Morris, Robert. *Family Responsibility—Implications of Recent Demographic and Service Trends for a Natural Helping System*. National Technical Information Service, U.S. Department of Commerce, 1977.
McGreehan, Deirdre M. and Warburton, Samuel W. "How to Help Families Cope With Caring for Elderly Members." *Geriatrics*, 33 (June 1978), 99-106.
National Retired Teachers Association, American Association of Retired Persons and Wakefield Washington Association, *Family Support Systems and The Aging—A Policy Report*, 1980.
Powers, Edward A.; Klith, Patricia; and Gondy, Willis. "Family Relationships and Friendships," in Robert C. Atchley (ed.), *Rural Environments and Aging*. Washington, D.C.: Gerontological Society, 1975, pp. 67-90.
Riley, Matilda W., et al. *Aging in American Society*. New York: Russell Sage Foundation, 1968.
Robertson, Joan F. "Grandparenthood: A Study of Role Conceptions." *Journal of Marriage and the Family*, 39 (February 1977), 165-174.
Robinson, Betsy and Thurnher, Majda. "Taking Care of Aged Parents: A Family Cycle Transition." *The Gerontologist*, 19 (December 1979), 586-593.
Savitsky, Elias and Sharkey, Harold. "The Geriatric Patient and His Family: Study of Family Interaction in the Aged." *Journal of Geriatric Psychiatry*, 5 (1, 1972), 3-19.
Seelbach, Wayne C. and Sauer, William J. "Filial Responsibility Expectations and Morale Among Aged Parents." *The Gerontologist*, 17 (December 1977), 492-499.
Shanas, Ethel. "Family-Kin Networks and Aging in Cross-Cultural Perspective." *Journal of Marriage and the Family*, 35 (August 1973), 505-511.
Shanas, Ethel. "The Family as a Social Support System in Old Age." *The Gerontologist*, 19 (April 1979), 169-174.

Shanas, Ethel and Sussman, Marvin B. *Family, Bureaucracy, and the Elderly*. Durham, N.C.: Duke University Press, 1977.
Shanas, Ethel. *The Health of Older People: A Social Survey*. Cambridge: Harvard University Press, 1962.
Shanas, Ethel and Streib, G. F. *Social Structure and The Family: Generational Relations*. Englewood Cliffs: Prentice-Hall, Inc., 1965.
Shanas, Ethel; Townsend, P.; Wedderburn, D.; Friis, H.; Milhoj, P.; and Stenhouwer, J. *Old People in Three Industrial Societies*. New York: Atherton Press, 1968.
Silverstone, Barbara. "Family Relationships of the Elderly." *Aged Care and Services Review*, 1 (March/April 1978), 3-9.
Simos, Bertha G. "Adult Children and Their Aging Parents." *Social Work*, 18 (May 1973), 78-85.
Streib, Gordon F. "Family Patterns in Retirement." *Journal of Social Issues*, 14 (2, 1958), 46-60.
Streib, Gordon F. "Older Families and Their Troubles: Familial and Social Responses." *The Family Coordinator*, 21 (January 1972), 5-19.
Sussman, Marvin B. "The Help-Pattern in the Middle-Class Family." *American Sociological Review*, 18 (February 1953), 22-28.
Sussman, Marvin B. "Relationships of Adult Children With Their Parents in the United States," in Ethel Shanas and Gordon F. Streib (eds.), *Social Structure and the Family: Generational Relations*. Englewood Cliffs, N.J.: Prentice-Hall, 1965, pp. 62-92.
Tibbitts, Clark. "Older Americans in the Family Context." *Aging* (April-May 1977), 8-11.
Townsend, Peter. "The Effects of Family Structure on the Likelihood of Admission to an Institution in Old Age: The Application of a General Theory," in Ethel Shanas and Gordon F. Streib (eds.), *Social Structure and The Family: Generational Relations*. Englewood cliffs, N.J.: Prentice-Hall, 1965, pp. 163-187.
Treas, Judith. "Family Support System for the Aged: Some Social and Demographic Considerations." *The Gerontologist*, 17 (December 1977), 486-491.
Troll, Lillian. "The Family of Later Life: A Decade Review." *Journal of Marriage and the Family*, 33 (May 1971), 263-290.
Troll, Lillian E.; Miller, Sheila; and Atchley, Robert C. *Families in Later Life*. Belmont, CA: Hadsworth Publishing Company, Inc., 1979.
Uhlenburg, Peter and Myers, Mary Ann. "Divorce and the Elderly." *Gerontologist*, 21 (June 1981), 276-282.
U.S. Bureau of the Census. *Statistical Abstract of the United States, 1981*. Washington, D.C., 1981.
U.S. Bureau of the Census. *Statistical Abstract of the United States, 1980*. Washington, D.C., 1980.
U.S. Comptroller General. Report to Congress. *The Well-Being of Older People in Cleveland, Ohio*. Washington, D.C.: U.S. General Accounting Office, 1977.
U.S. Congress, Senate, Special Committee on Aging. *Developments in Aging: 1980*, Part I, Report, 97th Cong., 1st Sess., 1981.
U.S. Congress, Senate, Special Committee on Aging. *Developments in Aging: 1981*, Vol. 1, Report, 97th Cong., 2nd Sess., 1982.
U.S. Congressional Budget Office. *Long-Term Care For Elderly and Disabled*. Washington, D.C.: U.S. Government Printing Office, February, 1977.
U.S. Department of Commerce, Bureau of Census. *Current Population Reports*. Special Studies, Series P-23, Number 84, 1979.
U.S. Department of Commerce, Bureau of the Census. *Current Population Reports*. Special Studies, Series P-20, No. 365, 1980.
U.S. Department of Health, Education, and Welfare, Public Health Services, Mental Health Administration. "Chronic Conditions and Limitations of Activity and Mobility, U.S., July 1955-June 1957." Public Health Service Publication No. 1,000, Series 10-61, Washington, D.C., January 1971.
U.S. Department of Health, Education, and Welfare. "Home Health Care for Persons 55

Years and Over." *Vital and Health Statistics Publication.* Statistics Publication Series, 10, No. 73, 1972.

Vinick, Barbara H. "Remarriage in Old-Age." *The Family Coordinator,* 27 (October 1978), 359-363.

Weeks, John R. and Cuellar, Jose B. "The Role of Family Members in The Helping Networks of Old People." *The Gerontologist,* 21 (August 1981), 388-394.

Wilson, Albert. "Family Life Among Elderly Persons," in Charles Crawford (ed.), *Health and the Family: A Medical-Sociological Analysis.* New York: Macmillan, 1971, pp. 22-23.

Wood, Vivian and Robertson, Joan F. "The Significance of Grandparenthood," in Jaber F. Gubrium (ed.), *Time, Roles, and Self in Old Age.* New York: Human Sciences Press, 1976, pp. 278-304.

Young, Ann M. "Work Experience of the Population in 1977." *Special Labor Force Report 224.* Washington, D.C.: U.S. Bureau of Labor Statistics, 1979.

Youmans, E. Grant. "The Rural Aged." *Annals of the American Academy of Political and Social Science,* 429 (January 1977), 81-90.

Chapter 3

Family Policy and Community-Based and In-Home Care for the Frail Elderly

A number of policy analysts have been concerned that public policies aimed at achieving family well-being be implemented. Kamerman and Kahn have noted that such a family policy should be concerned with ". . . both the effects on the family of all types of public activities and the efforts to use 'family well-being' as an objective, goal, or standard in developing public policy" (1976: 183). A public policy focus on family well-being has also been advocated by a number of other policy analysts (Moroney, 1976; Wynn, 1970; Winston, 1969; Moynihan, 1968; Myrdal, 1968; Rodman, 1968). As Moynihan has cautioned (1968: x):

> *A nation without a conscious family policy leaves to chance and mischance an area of social reality of the utmost importance, which in consequence will be exposed to the untrammeled and frequently thoroughly undesirable impact of policies arising out of other areas.*

A great deal of the literature on family policy is oriented to the care of children (Ross and Sawhill, 1976; National Research Council, 1976; Keniston and the Carnegie Council on Children, 1977; Fischman and Palley, 1978). However, recently this area has become a major concern for those interested in both the well-being of the functionally impaired elderly and the well-being and involvement of their caring relatives (Johnson and Bursk, 1977; Brody, Poulshock, and Maciocchi, 1978; Monk, 1979; Callahan et al., 1980; Schorr, 1980).

33

National Family Policy and the Elderly

Many of the economic, protective, educative, and recreational roles of the family have declined in modern industrial society in favor of, or in comparison with, the utilization of other social institutions. We believe that national policies should be developed in order to utilize the family to provide important protective, educative, and affectional roles for the chronically limited elderly. As Alva Myrdal (1968: 7) has commented:

Utilizing our knowledge and common sense we should reconsider in a realistic and cautious manner the division of functions between the family household and the national household and induce (through national policy) such changes in this division as may best preserve the fundamental values of our cultural heritage in a period of structural economic and social changes. Our social reforms should aim at conserving, not uprooting . . .

It is appropriate that a national family policy be directed toward the elderly. As we have shown, the large majority of the elderly are in close contact with family.

Existing national social programs provide meager support for family members caring for aged relatives, although several demonstration projects are underway in this area. These are discussed further in Chapter 6. (Most of these projects provide reimbursement under Medicare or Medicaid for services provided to the patient by family members.)

Current thinking about services for support of families caring for elderly relatives has been influenced by Litwak's work on relationships between formal organizations and primary groups. This work makes the assumption that primary groups such as families are best able to perform some functions (non-uniform, non-technical, unpredictable) and that bureaucracies best perform other tasks (uniform, technical, predictable) (Dobrof and Litwak, 1977). The implication of these assumptions is that in devising programs to support families, formal organizations have to find a balance which does not replace or discourage the family. The need is for flexible programs which build, wherever possible, on the strengths which families provide.

flexible → build on strength of family

Community-based programs for the chronically ill aged need to be developed with an understanding of the family unit. Such programs need not replace families as an institutional emphasis frequently does. Rather, they need to be designed carefully to complement the family's strengths, and to provide substitute services where families are not available. Families often need support which will enable them to fulfill responsibilities that they want to accept concerning dependent elderly members. Current programs such as tax credit programs, social security, SSI, health benefit programs, and social service programs need to be examined from the point of view of utilizing the family unit. The social policy goal should be to encourage, and not to punish or ignore, the families who choose to care for elderly relatives in need of long-term care.

Chronic Illness, Delivery of Services, and Appropriateness of Care

As previously mentioned, patterns of reduced fertility and advances in medical science (e.g., antibiotics) have resulted in an increase in the proportion of the aged in the general public, especially those in the 75 and over category. As medical science has controlled most of the acute illnesses which were prime causes of morbidity at the turn of the century, chronic diseases are now the major diagnoses of persons over 65 years of age. Chronic illness is characterized by gradual onset and progressive degeneration. It is very difficult, or in some instances impossible, to treat and is of lifelong duration. Chronic conditions include heart disease, arthritis, diabetes, some cancerous conditions, and visual or hearing defects.

According to the National Center for Health Statistics, 81 percent of persons 65 and older have at least one chronic condition, and many suffer from several chronic problems. Forty-five and one-half percent of the chronically ill elderly have activity limitations and 34.9 percent have major activity limitations.

Chronic conditions require different patterns of health care utilization than care for acute illness (LaVor, 1977). As Brody has observed (1979: 1870):

> The nature of chronic impairment implies a deficit over a period of time. An episodic response is ineffective and inappropriate to the need for rehabilitation. Instead continuity of care is necessary, a spectrum of services provided by a variety of disciplines and professions . . . whose collective goal is the

maintenance and improvement of the individual's level of functioning.

Thus, the acute-illness medical model is inadequate for dealing with the needs of the chronically ill. These needs are social, psychological, economic, and medical. Chronic conditions result in limited functioning which often affect an individual's sense of self-esteem and well-being. The chronically ill person often is less able to earn a living and to engage in social activities. Such persons are often unable to meet basic needs, such as shopping, housekeeping, cooking, eating, bathing, and dressing. High medical expenses, plus inflation and decreased earnings lead to impoverishment. What appears to be necessary to meet the needs of chronically limited persons and supportive families is a broad range of services to meet a complex set of interrelated needs. Such services range far beyond the medical area to include homemaker, personal care, transportation, counseling, recreational, social services, and financial support for home modification (Gross-Andrew and Zimmer, 1978; U.S. Congress, Senate, Committee on Energy and Commerce, 1981: 20-21). Families caring for relatives with mental confusion need companions or escorts. Such services should ideally be adequate, accessible, and well-coordinated.

Unfortunately, community-based services currently available to the chronically ill elderly in the United States fall far short of these goals.[1] Such services are certainly not uniformly available on a national basis. Available health services are skewed towards treatment of acute rather than chronic illness. Also, long-term care programs for the elderly have emphasized the nursing home as a focal point of services—rather than the delivery of home health and social care services.

Institutional Care: The Ascension of Nursing Home Care[2]

The ascendency of nursing homes rather than community-based long-term care in public policy started in the 1950s. When the 1956 Social Security amendments increased federal support for Old Age Assistance (OAA) and other assistance programs, they also established separate provision for vendor payments. Such states as New

---

[1]See Chapter 6 for an analysis of this problem.

[2]This section primarily relies upon Vladeck, 1980: 30-70.

York and Massachusetts substantially expanded vendor payments
for nursing home care at that time. Also, under the Hill-Burton program, a 1954 amendment provided for grants to public and non-
profit institutions for the construction of nursing homes. Vladek
notes that this was due to the interest group lobbying of the American Nursing Home Association (ANHA)—a group representing proprietary interests which sought federal funding for the financing of
capital costs. The Eisenhower Administration and Congress,
however, would only agree to financing of public, non-profit nursing homes operated in conjunction with hospitals. Medical Assistance for the Aged (MAA), a welfare measure passed in 1960, gave
another significant impetus to vendor payments for nursing home
services. Such vendor payments rose to $449 million, an approx-
imately 10-fold increase between 1960 to 1965. Thus prior to the
enactment of Medicare and Medicaid in 1965, public funds were
paying for an increasing share of nursing home costs.

While Medicare provides some reimbursement for a limited
period for skilled nursing home care, after the issuance of its 1969
Intermediary Letter 371 which listed such required skilled nursing
services as intraveneous feeding and injections, Medicare reimbursement has played a very limited role in the nursing home area.
Medicaid which allows federal-state reimbursement to nursing
home vendors—as a Medicaid required service in the case of Skilled
Care Facilities (SCFs) which provided round the clock nursing services and as an optional service in the case of Intermediate Care
Facilities (ICFs). (The ICFs are facilities in which patients are
viewed as needing less intensive medical care.) Such facilities
(SNFs and ICFs) were under Public Law 92-603 (1972) to be paid
on a reasonable cost related basis. Regulations implementing this
provision did not go into effect until January 1, 1978. (This requirement is eliminated by the Omnibus Reconcilation Act of 1981
[Public Law 97-35].) By 1979, 20,185 nursing homes with
1,407,000 beds were directly involved in providing services to
needy individuals. In 1980, expenditures for nursing home care services totaled $20.7 billion. Medicaid governmental payments ac-
counted for over half of such expenditures (U.S. Congress, Senate,
Special Committee on Aging, 1982: 355; Gibson and Waldo, 1981:
20 and 42). Such expenditures are divided between ICFs and SCFs.
States vary wildly in their proclivity to utilize primarily ICFs or
SNFs. California and Connecticut mainly use SNFs, Texas and
New Jersey mainly utilize ICFs, and Michigan predominantly

utilizes SNFs, but makes substantial use of ICFs (U.S. Health Care Financing Administration, 1979: 46-47).

Medicaid established a health and social service system for the frail elderly and others with chronic physical or mental limitations based primarily on the utilization of nursing homes. This process occurred reflexively, in an unplanned manner. While a primarily nursing home care approach to dealing with the chronically limited needs reassessment and refocusing in terms of increasing utilization of community-based approaches, it is politically difficult to achieve this end. Vladeck states (1980: 246) that:

> Dissatisfaction with public performance breeds immobility. That ideological process is closely linked to a balance of political forces. A political system characterized by multiple independent veto powers is much less likely to remove benefits previously conferred than it is to confer new ones. No one is very happy with prevailing policies which are themselves the product of past mistakes, but no one is able to do much about them either. Incrementalism is both a policy style and a political outcome, and these two characteristics continually feed on one another.

Institutional Care Versus Family Centered Care

Thus, a dimension of current public social policy which we are emphasizing in this analysis is that federal health programs for the elderly are generally oriented to an institutional approach. Government support for care for chronically ill elderly emphasizes the utilization of nursing homes rather than the adaptation of a significant community care focus.

A 1977 Congressional Budget Office (CBO) study estimated that of the 5-9.9[3] million functionally disabled, only 1.9-2.7 received help from any government program; 3-6.7 million received help from families, and .8-1.4 million received no long-term care at all. The study estimated that the ratio of non-institutionalized personal care services to institutional services is approximately one-and-a-half to one; 2.5 million non-institutionalized persons served in *comparison with* 1.7 million institutionalized persons served. A 1978

---

[3]This figure is not limited to the elderly, however, the elderly compose the most substantial part of this figure.

report of the Department of Health, Education, and Welfare's Long Term Care Task Force estimated that between 3.6 and 7.8 million individuals may be receiving long-term care services at home from family or friends or making do individually (U.S. Congress, Senate, Committee on Energy and Commerce, 1981: 2). It is clear that public program support of the family's role in long-term care could be substantially increased (U.S. General Accounting Office, 1977).

Moreover, according to the Congress Budget Office (1977) between 10 and 40 percent of the elderly in nursing homes could be cared for by community-based services. In spite of the extensive role of the family in the provision of long-term care for the chronically ill elderly, government programs emphasize services for individual patients in an institutional setting, which all but ignores the role of the family. Indeed such care often substitutes for possible alternative care which might be provided by family members.

In the Medicaid program emphasis on care for frail elderly persons is placed on long-term institutional placement, in spite of the fact that the physical, social, and psychological needs of many functionally impaired elderly persons are often not best served by such institutional arrangements. A decision to place an ill, elderly person in a nursing home may relate to the stress faced by family members in providing care to a chronically debilitated elderly relative. A New York study indicated that such stress may be a key factor in the decision to place an elderly relative in a nursing home, even though that facility is considered an undesirable choice (Brody, 1979: 1830).

Also, Medicaid program expenditures are heavily weighted to institutional arrangements. In calendar 1980, Medicaid benefits totaled $25.3 billion. The federal share of such personal health expenditures was 55 percent (Gibson and Waldo, 1981: 48). Medicaid payments were heavily institutional—41 percent of Medicaid payments went to nursing homes (over $10.3 billion) and 37.5 percent of payments went to hospitals (over $9.5 billion). Nine percent of payments were made to physician's services ($2.3 billion) and medically related home health service—was only one service included under the general rubric of "other health services." Expenditures in this latter category were $800 million or slightly more than three percent of Medicaid expenditures (Gibson and Waldo, 1981: 48). Thus, medically related home health expenditures under Medicaid, in spite of some recent increases, have been negligible in comparison with expenditures for nursing homes.

Institutionalization is also encouraged by the lack of adequate community-based alternatives. The discharge unit in the hospital generally finds it much easier to place a patient in a nursing home than to locate and activate an alternative complex network of community-based services which would be needed. Often considerable effort must be expended in locating an adequate community-based long-term care alternative, and then if just one needed service cannot be managed (e.g., transportation) the entire plan collapses.

The current emphasis on institutional care is unfortunate as most older persons are loathe to willingly choose this option. They wish to remain independent as long as possible and turn to family, friends, or community-based options such as boarding homes if they become functionally limited (Brickner, 1976; Shanas, 1960). Indeed, this is what usually happens. A comparison of the institutionalized and non-institutionalized elderly has shown that those in nursing homes are generally people who have limited family resources and/or are in the most severely disabled group; seven percent of the elderly in the community are extremely impaired and 76 percent of those in institutions are so impaired (Pfeiffer, 1976). It has been a matter of broad consensus that 15-25 percent of those in institutions could be maintained in the community if adequate support were available. This seems to be particularly feasible for people with mild levels of disability. However, recent studies do indicate that community-based care for a severely disabled individual with no family support would be very costly (U.S. General Accounting Office, 1977; Burton et al., 1974).

There has been increasing interest in community-based alternatives to institutional care, largely because the federal health-related programs (particularly Medicaid) have become so costly. Also, several studies have suggested that home care services can prevent a significant amount of institutionalization (Dunlop, 1976; Brickner et al., 1976; Neilson et al., 1972; Stassen and Holahan, 1981). Such home-based care may successfully rehabilitate elderly individuals who have suffered a chronic disability. Evaluation of such care in the Triage project, a Connecticut program emphasizing in-home and community-based services, indicated that among clients who survived through March 31, 1979, 32 percent of initial program participants had "improved or maintained their ability to carry out basic community living activities" such as meal preparation, housework, and shopping. Moreover between 25 and 30 percent of the Triage population was prevented from needing institutionalization as a result of receiving Triage services (U.S. Congress, Senate,

Committee on Energy and Commerce, 1981: 21). However, findings are not conclusive regarding cost savings or decreased rates of institutionalization where community-based alternatives are available. In a large study of day care and homemaker service programs authorized by Section 222 of the Social Security Amendments of 1972 (Weissert et al., 1980), the National Center for Health Services Research determined that reduction in cost due to decreased rates of institutionalization among the study populations were more than made up in program costs. In the homemaker group, rates of institutionalization were no lower than among the controls, but rates of hospital use were higher. However, both community-based programs examined seemed to result in lower death rates and higher contentment, improved functioning, and more social activity. Skellie et al. (1979) have also reported reduced death rates in populations receiving community-based service (alternative living services, day care, and home services).

Two studies indicate that home care is less expensive than institutional care at levels of mild and moderate disability, if family support is provided (U.S. General Accounting Office, 1977; Greenberg, 1974). However, for cases of severe disability nursing home cost is lower than home health and social service if costs to the family are considered.

It would be unfortunate if the studies we have noted were to lead to a continued emphasis on institutional care, since looking at cost alone overlooks the very important issues of quality of care and quality of life. In fact, there is widespread agreement in studies on community-based programs that these programs are more effective than institutions in improving or maintaining health, mental functioning, life satisfaction, and social activities (Doherty et al., 1978; Weissert et al., 1980; Gross-Andrew and Zimmer, 1978; Hodgson and Quinn, 1980).

Conclusion

Current policies which emphasize acute illness in home health programs, and institutional rather than community-based settings have contributed to an enormous gap in coverage of the long-term care needs for the chronically ill elderly. (As we will demonstrate in Chapter 5, current available home health service and other in-home services provided under a number of nationally funded programs often are inadequate in terms of being insufficient to meet the long-term care needs of the chronically ill elderly and are inequitable in terms of their fragmented and spotty availability.) At times, gaps have been filled by families. Because of the important role of the family in caring for the dependent elderly, policies need to place more emphasis on the family-based setting.

In view of the acute medical care service orientation of home care services under Medicare, and often under Medicaid, as well as the inability of current nationally funded health and social care programs to meet the community-based needs of many of the elderly with chronic conditions, a national family policy is essential with respect to the chronically ill elderly and caring relatives. Such a family policy should provide on a *systematic national basis* for a variety of community health and social services. The development on a national basis of systematic social service supports and ancillary health-functioning services should enable elderly individuals with chronic limitations to continue to function in the community and should assist concerned relatives who wish to maintain relationships with such elderly persons outside a custodial institutional setting wherever possible. Such a policy should de-emphasize the curative medical model for assisting the elderly in those situations in which it is an inappropriate model. Among the community health and social services which should be available to the chronically ill elderly as a matter of national family policy are physical rehabilitation aid in the community, visiting nursing, home health aide assistance, nurtitional assistance, as well as non-medically oriented long-term personal care, homemaker and chore services. Social services, which would include social work family service assistance (including counseling), should also be available to the chronically ill and concerned relatives. Finally, as child day care assists working parents, systematically available senior day care centers and respite care services would help the aged and assist concerned and involved children and other relatives. Also, a system of cash allowance or payment for services rendered would help families to provide home or community care for their elderly relatives. Other cash incentives could be made available to allow families to make structural alterations in existing homes in order to accommodate chronically ill elderly relatives.

Whatever the specific services or economic incentives provided, as a matter of national policy, it is important that they be designed in a highly flexible manner such that they will serve to build on the strengths of families rather than replacing the family's role in the support network.

REFERENCES

Burton, Richard M. et al. *Nursing Home Costs and Care: An Investigation of Alternatives.* Durham, N.C.: Duke University Center for the Study of Aging and Human Development, July 1974.

Brickner, Philip et al. "The Homebound Aged: A Medically Unreached Group." *Annals of Internal Medicine,* 82 (January 1975), 1-6.

Brody, Stanley J. "The Thirty-To-One Paradox: Health Needs of the Aged and Medical Solutions." *National Journal,* 11 (November 3, 1979), 1869-1873.

Brody, Stanley J.; Poulschock, S. Walter; and Masciocchi, Carla F. "The Family Caring Unit: A Major Consideration in the Long-Term Support System." *The Gerontologist,* 18 (December 1978), 556-561.

Callahan, James J., Jr.; Diamond, Lawrence D.; Giele, Janet Z.; and Morris, Robert. "Responsibility of Families for Their Severely Disabled Elders." *Health Care Financing Review,* 1 (Winter 1980), 29-48.

Dobrof, Rose; and Litwak, Eugene. *Maintenance of Family Ties of Long-Term Care Patients: Theory and Guide to Practice.* Washington, D.C.: U.S. Government Printing Office, 1977.

Doherty, Neville; Segal, Joan; and Hicks, Barbara. "Alternative to Institutionalization for the Aged: Viability and Cost Effectiveness." *Aged Care and Services Review,* 1 (January/February 1978), 1-8.

Dunlop, Burton. *Determinants of Long-Term Care Facility Utilization by the Elderly.* Washington, D.C.: The Urban Institute, March, 1976.

Fischman, Susan H.; and Palley, Howard A. "Adolescent Unwed Motherhood: Implications for a National Family Policy." *Health and Social Work,* 3 (February 1978), 30-46.

Gibson, Robert M.; and Waldo, Daniel R. "National Health Care Expenditures, 1980." *Health Care Financing Review,* 3 (September 1981), 1-54.

Greenberg, Jay. *Cost of In-Home Services.* Minneapolis, Minnesota: Governor's Council on Aging, 1974.

Gross-Andrew, Susannah; and Zimmer, Anna H. "Incentives to Families Caring for Disabled Elderly: Research and Demonstration Project to Strengthen the Natural Supports System." *Journal of Gerontological Social Work,* 1 (Winter 1978), 119-133.

Hodgson, Jr., Joseph H.; and Quinn, Joan L. "The Impact of the Triage Health Care Delivery System Upon Client Morale, Independent Living and Cost of Care." *The Gerontologist,* 20 (June 1980), 364-371.

Johnson, Elizabeth S.; and Bursk, Barbara J. "Relationship Between the Elderly and Their Adult Children." *The Gerontologist,* 17 (February 1977), 90-96.

Kamerman, Sheila B.; and Kahn, Alfred J. *Social Services in The United States.* Philadelphia: Temple University Press, 1976.

Keniston, Kenneth and The Carnegie Council on Children. *All Our Children: The American Family Under Pressure.* New York: Harcourt Brace Jovanovich, 1978.

LaVor, Judith. *Long-Term Care: A Challenge to Service Systems.* Washington, D.C.: U.S. Department of Health, Education, and Welfare, Office of Planning and Evaluation, September, 1976, Revised April 1977.

Monk, Abraham. "Family Supports in Old Age." *Social Work,* 24 (November 1979), 533-538.

Moroney, Robert M. *The Family and the State: Considerations for Social Policy.* New York: Longman, 1976.

Moynihan, Daniel P. "Forward to the Paperback Edition," pp. v-xvii, in Alva Myrdal, *Nation and Family*. Cambridge, Massachusetts: M.I.T. Press, 1978.

Myrdal, Alva. *Nation and Family*. Cambridge, Massachusetts: M.I.T. Press, 1968.

National Research Council, Advisory Committee on Child Development. *Toward A National Policy for Children and Families*. Washington, D.C.: National Academy of Sciences, 1976.

Nielson, Margaret; Blenkner, Margaret; and Bloom, Martin. "Older Persons After Hospitalization: A Controlled Study of Home Aide Service." *American Journal of Public Health*, 62 (August 1972), 1094-1101.

Pfiffer, Eric. *Multi-Dimensional Functional Assessment: The OARS Methodology*, 2nd Ed. Durham, North Carolina: Duke Center for the Study of Aging and Human Development, 1976.

Rodman, Hyman. "Family and Social Pathology in the Ghetto." *Science*, 161 (August 1968), 756-762.

Ross, Heather L. and Sawhill, Isabel V. *Time of Transition: The Growth of Families Headed by Women*. Washington, D.C.: The Urban Institute, 1975.

Schorr, Alvin. ". . . Thy Father and Thy Mother . . . " A Second Look at Filial Responsibility and Family Policy. Washington, D.C.: U.S. Department of Health and Human Services, Social Security Administration, 1980.

Shanas, Ethel et al. *Old People in Three Industrial Societies*. New York: Atherton, 1968.

Skellie, F. Albert; Coan, Ruth E.; and Jourdan, Louis F. "Community-Based Long-Term Care and Mortality: Impact One Year After Enrollment." Presented at American Public Health Association Annual Meeting, New York, NY, 1979.

Stassen, Margaret and Holahan, Joseph. Long-Term Demonstration Projects. *A Review of Recent Evaluations*. Washington, D.C.: The Urban Institute, February, 1981.

U.S. Congress, Congressional Budget Office. *Long Term Care for the Elderly and Disabled*. Washington, D.C., Government Printing Office, 1977.

U.S. Congress, Senate, Committee on Energy and Commerce. *Report on Experimental Efforts in Long-Term Care for the Elderly*, prepared for the Subcommittee on Health and the Environment, 97th Cong., 1st Sess., June 1981.

U.S. Congress, Senate, Special Committee on Aging. *Developments on Aging: 1981*, Vol. 1, *A Report of the Special Committee on Aging*, 97th Cong., 2nd Sess., February 22, 1982.

U.S. General Accounting Office. *Home Health—The Need for a National Policy to Better Provide for the Elderly*. Washington, D.C.: Government Printing Office, 1979.

Vladeck, Bruce C. *Unloving Care: The Nursing Home Tragedy*. New York: Basic Books, 1980.

Weissert, William G.; Wan, Thomas H.; and Livieratos, Barbara B. *Effects and Costs of Day Care and Homemaker Services for the Chronically-Ill: A Randomized Experiment*. Washington, D.C.: National Center for Health Services Research, February 1980.

Winston, Ellen. "A National Policy on the Family." *Public Welfare*, 27 (January 1969), 54-58.

Wynn, Margaret. *Family Policy*. London: Michael Joseph, 1970.

SECTION II

IN-HOME SERVICE PROGRAMS FOR THE CHRONICALLY LIMITED ELDERLY: AN ANALYSIS OF NATIONAL POLICY

Chapter 4

Methodological Considerations in the Study of In-Home Services

In this chapter, we examine some of the problems inherent in the study of the needs of the disabled elderly—particularly their need for in-home services. In our analysis of services for the chronically limited elderly population, we make the assumption that programs should be both equitable and adequate. We begin this chapter with a discussion of the values underlying this position. This chapter also provides the basis for assumptions which are used in subsequent analysis. Assumptions about the proportion of the elderly population which is disabled, the number of those who could be expected to use in-home services, and the current level of these services are discussed.

VALUES IN IN-HOME SERVICES

There are a number of basic values which can be used to support expansion of in-home services for the impaired elderly. For example, home health and other in-home services can be justified on *utilitarian* grounds. In other words,

1. In-home services for the elderly should be provided because they will provide comparable benefits at lower cost by preventing or postponing institutionalization; or

2. In-home programs will free up family caregivers and thus (a) increase their productivity and (b) reduce their use of costly health services because of physical and mental illness related to the stress of caring for elderly relatives.

However, a primary focus on "efficiency" would not always lead to support for in-home services. We now recognize that in-home services are only less costly if the recipient is moderately impaired. Under conditions of extreme impairment, institutional care may be the less costly alternative. Are there other values or goals which would support the use of in-home services even if they were more costly?

Another value which would support in-home services is "freedom of choice." If we believe that people should be able to choose their environment, regardless of cost, most would prefer home care to institutional living arrangements. A problem here is that the "freedom of choice" of the individual may conflict with the "freedom of choice" of the family. What happens when the elderly man chooses to live and be cared for by his daughter and she does not accept?

Other values which become entangled in arguments surrounding in-home services for the frail elderly relate to "families" and "communities." In many parts of American society, the ultimate value would be to maximize the role of these institutions.

While it is clear that these three types of justification can conflict in specific instances, the fact is that all three can be used to support a greater emphasis on in-home services. Today, a decision to expand in-home services would frequently increase individual choice, provide support for families, and reduce cost.

The issue is complicated, however, by the fact that the resources which support health and social services are limited. Where should the money to support expanded in-home services come from? Should in-home service be supported at the expense of institutional care or acute care services? Is the current emphasis on acute care justified because those in need of acute care have the potential to become functional, contributing members of society while those in need of chronic care frequently do not? Support for institutional care could be justified as a way of insuring that limited resources are channeled to those most in need.

The same type of dilemmas exist within the in-home service area. How do we insure that we are providing the most appropriate service given the degree of disability of the recipient? Should we channel all of the resources to those whose needs are most immediate (as Medicare tries to do by limiting its funding to acute needs), or should we provide a very minimal level of service to a large number of persons (as Title XX programs do)? This second alternative runs the risk of providing service at a level so low as to be meaningless.

An example would be a program which chooses to serve one meal a week to 210 people rather than three meals a day to 10 people. The one meal a week would not prevent the starvation of those who have no other way to get meals. Both alternatives may be viewed as inadequate: one meal a week is inadequate on a vertical level, while three meals a day for only a few of the needy is inadequate on a horizontal level.

In our analysis, we examine support programs for the disabled elderly with respect to "equity" and "adequacy." We assume, then, that a social service program should be equitable. In other words, it *should* be equally accessible to all at the same level of need. Secondly, we assume that service *should* be available at a level sufficient to meet the need. All disabled elderly should be *entitled* to a full range of services necessary to meet their respective needs—regardless of their economic status.

We do not argue that in-home services are necessarily always less costly than nursing home care, or that these services will make people economically productive. Nor do we consider the alternative uses of the funds which would be needed to meet this goal. This type of consideration is beyond the scope of this book. Instead, we merely acknowledge that our analysis is based on assumptions about the value of equitable and adequate service as an appropriate goal for a humane society. Additionally, we believe that maintaining frail elderly persons in a "least restrictive" environment appropriate to their conditions is a humane and desirable social goal.

MEASUREMENT OF ADEQUACY AND EQUITY

Any discussion of "adequacy" poses problems of definition. An "adequate" program must meet some standard based on a judgment of amount of service needed by a targeted group. Determination of program adequacy is complicated by the fact that different people may have different standards. Who is to define adequacy? the individual receiving the service? the family of that individual? the provider? the agency? the government? Each of these entities may have a different way of determining adequacy. Factors which might be very important to the individual (e.g., whether he/she likes the homemaker's cooking) may be immaterial to the agency or the government, which may be more concerned with the homemaker's technical qualifications.

A related issue, that of utilization, also complicates the determination of adequacy. It is conceivable that an individual will reject a service which a professional assesses him or her to need. Is administratively determined service *availability* enough to determine adequacy, or is service utilization required? In our subsequent analysis of in-home services, our estimate of adequacy is admittedly limited. We assume that service is adequate if 50 percent of the targeted population receives the service. With the data available, we are not able to consider the *quality* of the service, or even the *amount* of service. It is hoped that in the future more complete data will make more precise definitions of adequacy possible.

We define equity on an interstate basis, rather than on an individual state basis. In other words, we consider a program equitable if the same proportion of the target population receives service in all states. Because of the inadequacy of available data, we are not able to examine regional within-state differences, urban/ rural differences, or demographic differences such as socioeconomic status, ethnic or racial identity, sex or living arrangement. Again, it is hoped that the problems encountered in our limited analysis might illustrate the need for more detailed and systematic collection of data in this field.

MEASUREMENT OF NEED

Levels of Disability in the Elderly

In order to determine the adequacy of in-home service programs, some estimate of ''need'' is necessary. The first step in such a definition involves a determination of level of disability. In other words, it can be reasonably assumed that an individual who is functioning normally will be able to take care of his or her own personal care and housekeeping needs, and that home visits by medical personnel such as nurses, nurses aides, physical therapists, and social workers will not be necessary. However, definition and measurement of ''disability'' in the population is an area fraught with problems. First, consider how disability should be measured. The most traditional way is to depend on the judgment of trained clinicians (e.g., physicians). This method results in diagnosis of specific disease entities. For example, the physician may judge that an individual has arthritis or congestive heart failure. Thus, it is possible to estimate rates of these disease entities in the elderly population. However, there are several questions concerning use of clinical judgment to estimate levels of disability. The major problem is that within any single diagnosis there is a wide range of functional variations. Thus two people with the same diagnosis, say, cerebrovascular accident or stroke, might function at very different levels. Because of this variation, it would be impossible to equate certain diagnoses with certain levels of disability. To say, for example, that a stroke results in greater disability than arthritis, would not always be true. Another problem is that many elderly have more than one chronic condition, so that looking at rates of individual diseases would greatly over-estimate numbers of disabled. Finally, use of clinical assessment is impractical, as it is very costly.

While clinical measures may be good indicators of need for clinical medical services, they are not adequate to indicate needs for in-home services. Need for homemaker service, for example, would relate more to an individual's ability to perform housework than to the presence of a specific disease. Whether someone *actually* performs housework could also relate to mental capacity, presence of psychiatric problems, self-esteem, motivation, and/or previous roles in addition to physical capacity. Finally, the environment may or may not make this task necessary. Thus, measures of functioning are preferred to clinical diagnoses for predicting need for in-home services.

What information do we have, then, which would help us to estimate the proportion of the elderly population who are functionally disabled? Unfortunately, there have been very few national studies of disability.

Also, most of those interested in estimating or measuring disability are interested in persons whose disability prevents them from working. Thus, many of the measures of disability focus on the population of 18-64 years and depend on questions like "Do you have any health problem which keeps you from working?" These questions greatly underestimate disability in an elderly population— where a person might answer "no" because—although he or she has a disability, it does not prevent working because the person is already retired. (Studies by the Social Security Administration such as the Survey of Disabled Adults, and the disability questions included in the 1970 Census tend to be of this type.)

Most of our knowledge of disability in the elderly at the national level comes from the Health Interview Survey (HIS) which is a part of the National Health Survey conducted by the National Center for Health Statistics. The survey asks a number of questions about "activity limitation" which, as just mentioned, are problematic when applied to non-working populations, such as the elderly. More useful to us are the questions about mobility limitation. These questions indicate that 11.8 percent of the population 65 and over was either "confined to the house" or "needs help getting around." This figure is low from the point of view of need for in-home services, because there are many people who may be able to get around, but who still need help with housework, personal care, or nursing care. It is also not necessarily based on an interview directly with the disabled person. Therefore, it tends to underestimate levels of disability (The Urban Institute, 1975).

The other national study which has been widely used to estimate disability was done at Ohio State University (OSU) (Nagi, 1975). Like the HIS survey, this study did not focus on the elderly, but covered all age ranges. Because the sample size was only 5,000, this means that the number of disabled elderly was less than 200 persons—a very small number on which to estimate a population of several million. One of the measurements used in this study was a "scale of independent living." According to this survey, the proportion of the elderly population who needed assistance with mobility and/or personal care was 16.8 percent (see Table 1).

The numbers from these two national studies are not inconsistent since the definition of disability in the OSU study was broader than that in the HIS study. Neither, however, is broad enough to cover all those in need of in-home services.

Table 1 also shows the results of several studies which are geographically limited. These studies, however, have the advantage of (1) focusing on the target population, and (2) much more detailed measurement of functional disability. Surveys of about 1,000 elderly persons were conducted in Durham, North Carolina and Cleveland, Ohio. The OARS (developed by the Older Americans Resources and Services Group at Duke University) scale was applied. This is a multi-functional rating scale which combines measurements of impairment in five areas: social resources, economic resources, mental health, physical health, and activities of daily living (ADL) (capacity to perform various instrumental and physical tasks necessary for independent living). Moderate impairment in two or more functions was found in 20-22 percent of the elderly population. Unfortunately, because the different types of impairments create needs for different services, it is difficult to interpret these figures. In other words, it would be important to know whether the impairment was physical or economic in order to relate impairment to service needs. However, there was an attempt made in the Cleveland study to correlate services received with impairment levels. In this analysis, the five functional levels were combined into one impairment scale with eight intervals which range from Unimpaired to Extremely Impaired.[1] Only the Extremely Impaired (7 percent of the Cleveland elderly) were using skilled nursing service. Personal care services were used by the Extremely Impaired as well as the Greatly Impaired (a total of 14 percent of the population). Homemaker services were used by these persons as well as the Generally Impaired, the Moderately Impaired, and the Mildly Impaired, together adding another 44 percent (U.S. Comptroller General, 1978). Unfortunately, the report is not specific enough to determine what proportion of those in each impairment category needed the service. Again, because the impairment scores from the five dimensions are combined, it is difficult to draw implications for service from the results. Thus, the results are only broadly suggestive.

More recent work from Framingham, Massachusetts (Branch and Jette, 1981) provides measures of disability directly related to specific functions. The authors found 21 percent of those 65-74 years unable to perform housework, while among those 75-84 years, the figure was 36 percent (Table 1). In the same study (Jette and Branch, 1981), 29 percent of those 65-74 were considered unable to perform heavy housework, with the figure of 50 percent for those 75-84.

Finally, Table 1 shows that in a survey of the elderly covering the State of Massachusetts, 6 percent can be defined as "vulnerable." In this study, the definition of vulnerable involved either having three or more unmet needs for social services or making extensive use of health services. This definition would describe an especially needy subset of the population which uses in-home services.

What can be concluded from the data in Table 1? First, it is obvious that there is presently no simple answer to the question of how to identify the disabled elderly population. Various studies of "disability" have defined disability differently, depending on the

[1]This terminology has been previously discussed in Chapter 2.

TABLE 1: Major Studies Which Estimate the Extent of Disability in the Elderly

Author	Date	Location	Sample	Definition of "Elderly"	Measurement	Definition of "Disability"	Percent of Elderly Population Disabled
Nagi, Saad Ohio State Univ. (a)	1972	USA	5,000 persons over 18 years	65+	Independent Living Index	Percent who need mobility assistance and/or personal care assistance	16.8%
National Center for Health Statistics (b)	1972	USA	persons of all ages	65+	Household interviews; HIS indicators due to chronic conditions	Confined to the house or needs help getting around	11.8%
Duke Center for the Study of Aging and Human Development (c)	1973	Durham County North Carolina	990 elderly persons residing in the community (non-institutionalized)	65+	OARS (household interviews)	Moderate impairment or worse in two or more functions	22%
U.S. General Accounting Office (c)	1975	Cleveland, Ohio	1,069 elderly persons residing in the community (non-institutionalized)	65+	OARS (household interviews)	Moderate impairment or worse in two or more functions	20%

(a) Saad Z. Nagi. "An Epidemiology of Adulthood Disability in the United States." Mershon Center, Ohio State University, 1975 (unpublished).

(b) U.S. Department of Health, Education, and Welfare, National Center for Health Statistics. Limitations of Activities and Mobility Due to Chronic Conditions, United States, 1972. Series 10, Number 96, U.S. Government Printing Office, Washington, D.C., 1974.

(c) Multidimensional Functional Assessment: The OARS Methodology; A Manual. Duke University Center for the Study of Aging and Human Development, Durham, North Carolina, 1978.

TABLE 1: Continued

Author	Date	Location	Sample	Definition of "Elderly"	Measurement	Definition "Disability"	Percent of Elderly Population Disabled
Branch, Laurence G. (d)	1976	Massachusetts	1,317 non-institutionalized elderly	65+	Personal Interviews. Combination of unmet needs for social service and level of health care utilization	Persons who had three or more unmet needs for social service or made extensive use of health care services were defined as "vulnerable"	6%
Branch, Laurence G. and Jette, Alan M. (e) Howard Medical School	1976–1978	Framingham, Massachusetts	2,654 surviving members of the cohort from the Heart Disease Epidemiological Study	65-84	Need for assistance with housekeeping, food preparation and grocery shopping Personal or telephone interviews	Percent who experience difficulty performing this function. Includes those whose need for assistance is met as well as those whose need is unmet.	Housekeeping 65-74 yrs - 21% 75-84 yrs - 36% Food Preparation 65-74 yrs - 18% 75-84 yrs - 14% Grocery Shopping 65-74 yrs - 5% 75-84 yrs - 17%
Jette, Alan M. and Branch, Laurence (f) Howard Med. School	1976–1978	Framingham, Massachusetts	2,654 surviving members of the cohort from the Heart Disease Epidemiological Study	65-84	Rosow and Breslaw's Functional Health Scale	Percent reporting inability to perform heavy household work	65-74 yrs - 29% 75-84 yrs - 50%

(d) Laurence G. Branch. Vulnerable Elders. Gerontological Monograph, Gerontological Society, Washington, D.C. 1980.

(e) Laurence G. Branch and Alan M. Jette. "The Framingham Disability Study: I. Social Disability Among the Aging." American Journal of Public Health, 71 (November 1981), 1202-1210.

(f) Alan M. Jette and Laurence G. Branch. "The Framingham Disability Study: II. Physical Disability Among The Aging." American Journal of Public Health, 71 (November 1981), 1211-1216.

goal of the study. Studies designed to estimate the need for services of the elderly population are recent and suffer from several problems. One is that they are not national. Those which are national in scope tend to be studies in which a few questions on disability are added to a long questionnaire designed for a broader purpose. These do not produce the precise information on levels of disability needed for predicting needs for services. Secondly, the local studies vary considerably in the way disability or need for service is measured. Even when the same measure is used in several studies (as with the OARS in recent years) the results are often presented in an aggregated way which make cross-survey comparisons difficult or impossible.

It is also clear from the various studies of disability that there is a wide range of "disability" in the population, from persons who are bedridden to those who are only mildly impaired. Arriving at any one figure for proportion of the elderly population which is disabled involves setting some arbitrary cut-off point on the continuum. Where would such a cut-off be set when the goal is to determine needs for in-home services? The General Accounting Office's (GAO) Cleveland data suggest that about 7 percent need skilled nursing. Those who are bedridden, who need help with personal care or with mobility could also be expected to need in-home services. The data in Table 1 would suggest that this population would comprise 12-17 percent of the elderly population. However, this cut-off may be too severe. Studies on the need for household help suggest the proportion may be in the 20-35 percent range. Thus, the numbers in need depend on the specific type of in-home service, and range from 7-35 percent.

In Chapter 5, when we examine the adequacy of in-home services on a state-by-state basis, we use the figure of 18 percent to estimate the number of disabled elderly in each state. Clearly, this is an arbitrary figure. However, it is a conservative estimate, which can be supported from the data on levels of disability and which will not set an exaggerated standard that no state can meet.

Before continuing this discussion, it is important to emphasize the need for more careful research which relates specific functional levels to the need for specific types of service. This should be done with much finer measurements than are typically used to measure function. Also, the need for service should be clearly specified. "Is household help needed daily, weekly, or once a year?" "How much help is needed?" etc. This research should also examine sociodemographic characteristics and how they relate to func(well as regional variation. Such data collection should be and national in scope.

ESTIMATING NEED FOR IN-HOME SERVICES

While we have a rough estimate of the size of the elderly population who are disabled to the point of not being able to perform certain functions, we must be careful not to equate levels of disability with need for service from a public program. There are several reasons for this. First, as discussed in Chapter 2, many of the needs of the disabled elderly are being met by informal sources such as family members. Some of the disabled elderly who do not receive service from family members may be able to purchase services from proprietary agencies or providers. Finally, some disabled elderly would reject in-home services from any public program even if they were not able to obtain the services from private resources. This could be due to pride, dissatisfaction with the service available, etc. For these reasons, we would expect that levels of expressed need for service would be lower than levels of disability in any population. The question remains: How can we estimate how much lower?

Unfortunately, there is very little data available which can be used to make this estimate. One relevant piece of information which comes from the GAO Cleveland study (U.S. General Accounting Office, 1977) is that home help services are highly acceptable to the elderly population. About 80 percent of those who were unable to perform housework expressed a need for household help. (This is much higher than for services such as mental health or financial counseling.)

Another indication that utilization of in-home services is potentially quite high among the disabled elderly comes from the experience of several recent demonstration programs which have made in-home services easily available to their target populations (see Table 2). While these programs are described in more detail in Chapter 5, here we are looking only at the utilization of in-home services. We find a range from 35 percent (Triage) to 86 percent Natural Supports Program (NSP). Again, there are problems in interpreting this data. First, although all of the programs were available only to disabled elderly, the definitions of disability in the different programs varied greatly. Secondly, the services available

TABLE 2: Utilization of Various In-Home Services in Demonstration Programs

Study	Date	Location	Population	Results
Wisconsin Community Care Organization (a)	1977	Milwaukee, Wisconsin	187 cases, Medicare eligibles with Geriatric Functional Rating Scale scores of 20 or less	13% - Home Health Aides 46% - Personal Care 52% - Home Management Services
Natural Supports Project (b)	1981	New York City	96 cases, Functionally disabled, 60+ low income and with natural support	86% - Homemaker Services (includes personal care)
Community Care Program (c)	1979	Illinois	Over 7,000 cases, 60+ and "in danger of premature or unnecessary institutionalization."	60% - Used Chore/ Homemaker Services
Triage (d)	1982	Connecticut	2,623 persons 65+, at high risk for institutionalization	34% - Visiting Nurses 16% - Home Health Aide 18% - Homemaker

(a) Robert Applebaum, Frederick W. Seidl, and Carol D. Austin. "The Wisconsin Community Care Organization: Preliminary Findings from the Milwaukee Experiment." The Gerontologist, 20 (June 1980), 350-355.

(b) Dwight Frankfather, M.S. Smith, and Francis G. Caro. Family Care of the Elderly. Lexington, Ma: Lexington Books, 1981.

(c) Merlin S. Taber, S. Anderson, and C.J. Rogers. "Implementing Community Care in Illinois: Issues of Cost and Targeting in a Statewide Program." The Gerontologist, 20 (June 1980), 380-384.

(d) Joan L. Quinn. Triage II: Coordinated Delivery of Services to the Elderly. Wethersfield, Connecticut, 1982.

varied between the programs. Thus, it is hard to say if the differences in utilization among the programs reflected different service packages, different populations, or both. Estimating a specific rate of utilization, then, is difficult, although it is probably safe to say that it would fall between 35 and 85 percent of the disabled population.

Another type of data relevant to the question of the relationship between level of disability and need for public service is measurement of unmet need. A few studies have determined not only the respondent's ability to perform certain functions, but also whether his or her need for help is currently met. In Table 3, two such studies are presented. The General Accounting Office study, based on the OARS, found wide variation in level of need in different localities (25 percent needed help with ADL in urban Lane Co., Oregon, and fully 65 percent needed such help in rural Kentucky!).

TABLE 3: Levels of Unmet Need for In-Home Services

Study	Date	Location	Population	Proportion of Population in Need of Service	Proportion of Population With Unmet Need for Service
General Accounting Office (a)	1977	Cleveland, OH	1,311 persons 65+	41% could not perform daily tasks without help	21% were not receiving all the help they needed
		Lane Co., Oregon 1) Urban	318 persons 65+	25% could not perform daily tasks without help	14% were not receiving all the help they needed
		2) Town	124 persons 65+	32% could not perform daily tasks without help	18% were not receiving all the help they needed
		3) Rural	426 persons 65+	26% could not perform dialy tasks without help	15% were not receiving all the help they needed
		Rural, North-eastern KT	128 persons 65+	65% could not perform daily tasks without help	35% were not receiving all the help they needed
Branch and Jette (b)	1976-1978	Framingham, Massachusetts	2,654 surviving members from the Heart Disease Epidemiological Study, 65-84 years	23% had need for house-keeping help	6%: need met, potential problem 13%: uncertain need met, potential problem 4%: need unmet, current problem

(a)
Home Health -- The Need for a National Policy to Provide for the Elderly. Report to the Congress, Comptroller General, Washington, D.C. 1977, Enclosure I, page 9.

(b)
Laurence G. Branch and Alan M. Jette. "The Framingham Disability Study: I." American Journal of Public Health, 71 (November 1981), 1202-1210.

However, in all areas, the proportion whose needs remained unmet ran about 50 percent. The second study, conducted in Framingham, Massachusetts, found 23 percent could not perform housework, and thus needed housekeeping help. However, 19 percent were receiving adequate help and for only 4 percent (about one out of six) this need remained unmet. It is possible that the difference (4 percent compared to 50 percent) reflects the difference in the instrument used to measure unmet needs. It is also possible that there are real differences in resources available to the two populations. The Massachusetts group is of higher socio-economic status, and may be more able to purchase services to meet their needs. They also may have more family resources. Finally, the difference may reflect very real differences in the type of community services available in the two areas. Perhaps all of these factors are involved. Using current levels of unmet need to estimate need for public in-home services in the disabled elderly population is problematic because those needs now being met adequately by public programs are not included. Thus the level of need in the entire disabled population can be expected to be higher than the current level of unmet need.

Again, the data do not lead us to a clear answer to the problem of how to estimate need for services from disability levels. The relevant data available show wide ranges for both utilization and levels of unmet need. Clearly, research which uses a detailed, consistent instrument and systematic data collection techniques across all regions of the country, and which explores reasons for non-utilization of in-home services, is needed if we are to begin to unravel these problems. In Chapter 5, we will use the figure of 50 percent provision to the disabled elderly as an adequate level of in-home service provision. Again, this figure is arbitrary, but it represents a middle-range estimate considering the available data.

PROBLEMS IN ESTIMATING SERVICE
PROVIDED UNDER CURRENT PROGRAMS

One might think that, having defined an approximate level of disability (18 percent) and a proportion of the disabled who could be expected to use in-home services if available (50 percent), the determination of the adequacy of current programs would be relatively easy. A simple comparison between the number predicted to need these services and the number who actually receive them could be made. Unfortunately, the number of persons who receive in-home services is not always easy to determine. There are several reasons for this. First, there are a wide variety of programs which provide these services. As there is no central registry functioning (outside of the few demonstration programs where these services were coordinated), it is not possible to determine to what extent the populations of the different programs overlap. Also, there are no clear national guidelines for how figures should be tabulated, especially in the Federal-State programs (Medicaid, Title III, and Title XX). Since there is wide discrepancy between states on rates such as number of persons served and number of in-home visits provided, it is likely that different states count these items in different ways. Since total numbers receiving service are not cross-tabulated by visits, it is impossible to know if some states provide more service to fewer persons, or if it is just a question of a different criterion for inclusion in the number base. For example, if a visit by a social worker from the homemaker service is made for assessment purposes, and the service is not determined to be necessary, is this counted as a ''case'' or not? Justification could be developed either way, but that is not the point. What is needed is a clear set of guidelines which determine what numbers need to be reported and how they are to be compiled. Also, as mentioned earlier, a central registry of recipients of in-home services is also needed so that multiple service users could be identified to avoid double or triple counting. Because reporting of numbers served is often related to future funding, the reporting system needs to be separated from the fiscal process. Otherwise, agencies will be motivated to exaggerate their population base. Finally, some programs currently report quarterly, while others report annually. A quarterly figure cannot be converted into an annual figure by multiplying by four, because many clients can be expected to use the service over two or more quarters. Therefore, a consistent reporting system across states and across programs would not only mean consistent definitions, but also consistent time periods.

CONCLUSIONS

We would like to make note of a 1979 U.S. General Accounting Office report calling for a national information system for measuring the personal conditions of older people and for evaluating the services provided to them. The report observes:

To design and plan for the delivery of services to older persons, society, the Congress, and the executive branch need information on their well-being, the factors that make a difference in their lives, and the impact of services on them. Currently, this information is spread piecemeal throughout Federal, State, local, and private agencies. The result: Federal agencies have not evaluated the combined effect of these services, and in the absence of such information, assessing the impact of various laws on the lives of older people is difficult. (U.S. General Accounting Office, 1979: ii)

This report goes on to recommend that there should be established:

. . . a comprehensive national information system that determines the personal conditions of, problems of, and help available to older people . . . . The system should be expanded over time to include information necessary to study why older people do not receive the help they need and how family and friends can be encouraged to provide . . . help. (U.S. General Accounting Office, 1979: v)

Our study confirms the need for systematic collection of national data relating to the problems of the frail elderly and the availability of in-home and related community-based services for the frail elderly. In conclusion, we make the following recommendations:

Summary of Methodological Recommendations

1. Measuring Disability Levels
National research is needed which (1) uses a finely tuned instrument to measure functional limitation, (2) considers limitation specifically for elderly males and females as it relates to age appropriate roles and activities, (3) is longitudinal, (4) identifies relevant characteristics of aged cohorts so that we do not make the mistake of projecting today's disability level on tomorrow's elderly.

2. Measuring Need for In-Home Services
National research is needed which (1) differentiates need from unmet need, (2) differentiates those "able to benefit from" from those who express "need," (3) differentiates utilization

from "need," (4) accounts for differences in available services across localities and differences in accessibility within those localities, (5) is longitudinal, (6) correlates specific disability levels with needs for specific types of services and specific amounts of service, (7) correlates population characteristics with patterns of service utilization (given equal access).

REFERENCES

Applebaum, Robert; Seidl, Frederick W.; and Austin, Carol D. "The Wisconsin Community Care Organization: Preliminary Findings from the Milwaukee Experiment." *The Gerontologist,* 20 (June 1980), 350-355.

Branch, Laurence G. and Jette, Alan M. "The Framingham Disability Study: I. Social Disability Among the Aging." *American Journal of Public Health,* 71 (November 1981), 1202-1210.

Branch, Laurence G. *Vulnerable Elders,* Gerontological Monograph. Gerontological Society, Washington, D.C., 1980.

Duke University. *Multidimensional Functional Assessment: The OARS Methodology; A Manual.* Durham, North Carolina: Duke University Center for the Study of Aging and Human Development, 1978.

Frankfather, Dwight; Smith, M. S.; and Caro, Francis G. *Family Care of the Elderly.* Lexington, Ma.: Lexington Books, 1981.

Jette, Alan M. and Branch, Laurence G. "The Framingham Disability Study: II. Physical Disability Among the Aging." *American Journal of Public Health,* 71 (November 1981), 1211-1216.

Nagi, Saad Z. "An Epidemiology of Adulthood Disability in the United States." Columbus, Ohio: Mershon Center, Ohio State University, 1975. (Unpublished.)

Quinn, Joan L. *Triage II: Coordinated Delivery of Services to the Elderly.* Wethersfield, Connecticut, 1982.

Taber, Merlin S.; Anderson, S.; and Rogers, C. J. "Implementing Community Care in Illinois: Issues of Cost and Targeting in a Statewide Program." *The Gerontologist,* 20 (June 1980), 380-388.

The Urban Institute. *Report of the Comprehensive Needs Survey.* Washington, D.C., 1975.

U.S. Comptroller General. *The Well-Being of Older People in Cleveland, Ohio.* Washington, D.C., April 1977.

U.S. Comptroller General. *Home Health—The Need for a National Policy to Better Provide for the Elderly.* Washington, D.C., December 30, 1977.

U.S. Department of Health, Education, and Welfare, National Center for Health Statistics. *Limitations of Activities and Mobility Due to Chronic Conditions, United States, 1972.* Series 10, Number 96, U.S. Government Printing Office, Washington, D.C., 1974.

U.S. General Accounting Office. *Conditions of Older People: National Information System Needed.* Washington, D.C., 1979.

Chapter 5

The Level of Provision of Home Health and Other In-Home Services for the Chronically Limited Elderly: Some Considerations of Equity, Adequacy, and Public Accountability

As our population becomes increasingly older, the number of disabled elderly who remain in the community can be expected to increase. Such elderly persons often suffer from chronic diseases which, over time, come to interfere with daily functioning. In this chapter, we examine the structure of four major programs funding home health and/or other in-home services for the elderly with two types of questions in mind. First, we examine the extent to which these programs achieve horizontal equity (providing comparable services for consumers with comparable needs among different states) (Burns, 1965; Ozawa, 1974; Ozawa, 1978; Ozawa, 1982; Davidson, 1979; Palley and Palley, 1972; Palley and Palley, 1974; Palley, Palley, and Harkens, 1975). Secondly, we examine the extent to which adequate services were provided (the extent to which the programs provide sufficient benefits which meet the social and physical needs of consumers within different states). It is our hope that the answers to these questions will help policy makers to formulate programs which will best serve the needs of the community-based disabled elderly.

The scope of home health services is broad. Such services may include visiting nurse, health aide, personal care, physical therapy, equipment, and nutrition services. Other in-home services may include such homemaker/chore services as cooking, shopping, housework, laundry, and home repair, and such social services as counseling, advocacy, companionship, and transportation.

In this chapter, we focus primarily on home health services and homemaker services. Our analysis addresses problems of equity and adequacy regarding provision of such services in the following programs: Medicare, Medicaid, Title XX of the Social Security Act, and Title III of the Older Americans Act.

EQUITY WITHIN PROGRAMS

In this section, we will examine the extent to which the four major programs providing in-home services to the disabled elderly achieve within-program equity. That is, to what extent is the level of within program service provision comparable across the fifty states?

Discussion of Methodology

State program levels may reflect the fact that some states have much higher proportions of elderly persons in their populations than others. Administration on Aging data for 1977 show that four states (California, New York, Florida, and Pennsylvania) together had 30 percent of the nation's elderly. Eleven states had 58 percent of the nation's elderly population. By 1980, this location pattern had remained essentially unchanged (see Figure 1). Also, ten states had proportions of elderly substantially above the national average (see Figure 2). Therefore, before examining figures on numbers of recipients of in-home services, we take the size of the elderly population into account. However, only a minority of the elderly are disabled and potentially in need of such service. In this analysis, we make the assumption that the proportion of elderly who are disabled is the same for all states. Although estimates of disability vary, we will use the figure 18 percent to apply to all states.[1] For each state, then, a figure calculated as 18 percent of the number of persons aged 65 and over (1977 AOA figures) is used as an estimate of the

---

[1]There is no clear, widely accepted definition or measure of "disability" of the elderly. Instead, different studies have used different measures, or selected different cutting points on the continuum from healthy to extreme disability. Estimates of disability in those over 65 range from a low of 12 percent from the National Center for Health Services (NCHS) based on those who "need help getting around," to 17 percent (Nagi) "mobility and personal care assistance needed," to 23-26 percent from the General Accounting Office (GAO) "Generally, Greatly, or Extremely Impaired," based on the Older Americans Rating Scale (OARS). For a discussion of the Older Americans Rating Scale, see Pfeiffer, 1978; Nagi, 1975. For a discussion of the derivation of the above figure, see *supra.* Chapter 4.

FIGURE 1

POPULATION AGED 65 AND OLDER, TOP TEN STATES: 1980

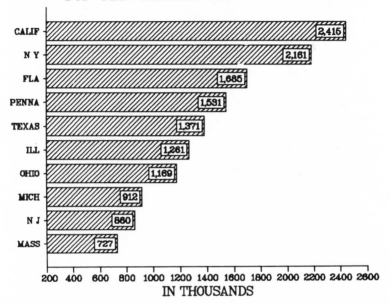

Source: U.S. Census of Population, 1980.

disabled elderly population in that state.[2] Numbers of recipients of in-home services are expressed as the number of recipients per thousand disabled elderly persons in the state. In this way, comparisons are made with respect to level of service between states of different sizes and with different sized elderly populations. We also have examined expenditure levels where disparities appear to relate to differential within program levels of service. To facilitate comparisons, all data used in this analysis are from 1977.

Medicare

Community-based services under Medicare involve home health and supportive services as ordered by a physician. Medicare, a

---

[2]The application of 18 percent to every state is arbitrary and needs to be interpreted cautiously. State-by-state variations in programs should be examined more closely in light of population characteristics.

FIGURE 2

PERCENTAGE OF TOTAL POPULATION AGED 65 AND OLDER, TOP TEN STATES: 1980

IN THOUSANDS

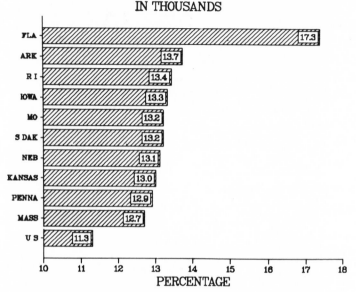

Source: U.S. Census of Population, 1980.

federally administered national program, provides health insurance benefits, most (90 percent) of which go to the elderly. At the time of this study, such benefits covered up to 100 home visits for home health care per illness under its hospital care provisions (Title 18A of the Social Security Act) and 100 visits per illness under its Supplementary Medical Insurance provisions (Title 18B). Part A services were preceded by a three-day hospital stay and a plan for such services was to be established within 14 days after discharge from a hospital or skilled nursing facility.[3] Service coverage under home health care titles includes some social services, intermittent nursing care, physical therapy, home health aide, and homemaker services (on an experimental basis) and medical equipment and supplies as ordered by a physician. Part B, Supplementary Medical Insurance home health services did not require a previous hospital stay.

Nationally, in terms of types of services received under the home

---

[3]These limitations were eliminated under 1980 Amendments to the Medicare legislation.

health care titles of Medicare, in 1977 over 660,000 beneficiaries (96 percent of persons served) received nursing care services; and home health aides served 224,000 persons (32.5 percent of persons served). While physical therapy services were received by 20 percent of patients, 4.6 million visits (30 percent of home health service visits) were by home health aides. Where such services were utilized, they were provided at a rate of 21 visits per person served.

Demographically, 58 percent of the persons served were age 75 and over and 93 percent had a status of aged under Medicare (65 and over). Seven percent received benefits under disability status or due to end-stage renal disease status.

In order to qualify for such home health service benefits, a beneficiary must be under the care of a physician, and be confined to his home. The physician must reach a determination of the patient's need for home health service. Thus, while Medicare provides for home health care services, these services were statutorily oriented to acute—quickly receding—conditions amenable to "cure" through skilled nursing care rather than to the supportive and long-term rehabilitative care needed by many chronically ill elderly. At the time of the study, such services were available only for a limited duration. It must also be noted that home health services make up a very small part of the total Medicare expenditures for the elderly. In 1977, total charges for Medicare home health services were only $407.8 million.

In 1977, the highest levels of services under the Medicare home health care titles were in Vermont (412 per 1,000 disabled elderly), Maine (286 per 1,000), Mississippi (263 per 1,000), New Hampshire (280 per 1,000), and Pennsylvania (257 per 1,000) (see Figure 3). The lowest Medicare home health care service levels were in the following eight states: North Dakota (36 per 1,000), Arkansas (53 per 1,000), Oklahoma (56 per 1,000), South Dakota (57 per 1,000), Kansas (61 per 1,000), Alaska (62 per 1,000), Indiana (67 per 1,000), and Iowa (68 per 1,000) (see Figure 3). Data are inadequate regarding the specific nature of such services. However, an overall pattern of inequity in terms of the availability of service levels between the states is demonstrated.

The same pattern of inequity is evident in the Medicare reimbursement for home health care services for 1977 (over $354.5 million).[4] Over 30 percent of this amount went to three states—New

---

[4]The subsequent analysis utilizes U.S. Department of Health, Education, and Welfare, Health Care Financing Administration, 1977.

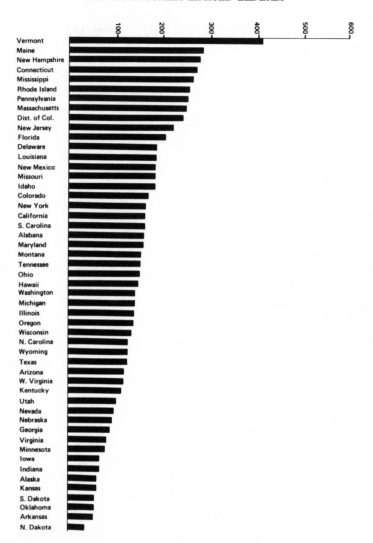

FIGURE 3. Number of Recipients of Home Health Services under Medicare per 1,000 Disabled Elderly, 1977.

York, Florida, and California—which together constitute slightly less than 25 percent of the targeted elderly population. At the other end of the spectrum, the eight states which were lowest in federal spending for Medicare home health services received 1.7 percent of federal spending, while the proportion of the disabled elderly living in these states was seven percent. These figures show a great deal of state-by-state variation in level of service and expenditure. This type of inequity is also apparent in Medicare home health statistics which show great regional variation in numbers served and charges. For example, per person charges in 1977 varied from $1,107 in Mississippi to $163 in South Dakota.[5]

One reason for inequity in relative levels of service is that receipt of home health services is very much dependent on the local health delivery infrastructure. Seventy-five percent of persons served by home health agencies lived in metropolitan areas. Such persons received 75 percent of total visits, accounting for 79 percent of visit charges. More than 29 persons per 1,000 enrolled in metropolitan areas received Medicare home health services while the rate for non-metropolitan area receipt of such services was under 20 per 1,000.

In sum, it is clear that while Medicare is a federally funded and administered program, it is essentially a vendor program which is dependent on the availability of local services and which funds at a locally prevailing charge basis. It is clear from the data presented that there were significant regional and local inequities between states and localities under the Medicare home health care titles. However, as we shall see, the inequities of Medicare were less severe than those of other federal programs which provide home health and other in-home services for the disabled elderly.

Medicaid

Home health services under Medicaid are defined as: "Services furnished to a patient in his home, including intermittent or part-time nursing service provided by a home health agency, or by a registered professional nurse, or licensed practical nurse, medical supplies, equipment, and appliances for use in the home, and services of a home health aide" (U.S. Department of Health, Education, and Welfare, Health Care Financing Administration, 1980). Every Medicaid program must provide home health services for individuals 21 years of age and older in those instances where such individuals are receiving federally supported, means tested financial assistance; such benefits may be provided optionally to other

---

[5]The data in this section are derived primarily from Callahan, 1977. Also, see U.S. Department of Health, Education, and Welfare, Health Care Financing Administration, undated b.

"medically needy" individuals. Eligibility for Medicaid may be achieved by participation in federally assisted welfare programs such as Aid to Families with Dependent Children (AFDC) and Supplementary Security Income (SSI) for the aged, blind, and disabled. Only one state, Arizona, does not participate in the Medicaid program. Generally, states must cover all federally assisted cash assistance recipients. The one exception is that states may exercise an option of limiting Medicaid coverage to recipients by requiring such recipients to meet a more restrictive standard of eligibility in effect on January 1, 1972, prior to the implementation of SSI. Fifteen states have exercised this option. States may also provide Medicaid coverage to those who are medically needy because high medical expenses have reduced their net income to that of the categorical groups of the needy aged, blind, disabled, or the AFDC family. Families whose incomes exceed 133-1/3 percent of the amount ordinarily paid to AFDC families are not eligible for the federal Medicaid program. Thirty-three states currently provide coverage for the medically needy. "Medically needy" implies a test of both medical need and limited financial capability to pay for services. Thus, Medicaid "by definition" does not seek to serve all the chronically ill elderly. It serves the chronically ill elderly only after they have exhausted their financial resources. Using our definition of equity, Medicaid by virtue of its state-by-state variations is inequitable in the sense of diverse state limitations on eligibility for services or availability of services.

In terms of the estimate of the number of disabled elderly in the population in comparison with the number of such persons receiving home health service from Medicaid, it appears that in fiscal 1977 (U.S. Department of Health, Education, and Welfare, Health Care Financing Administration, 1980) (if one makes the assumption that Medicaid home health services went mainly to the elderly) Connecticut's Medicaid program served 850 per thousand of the target group. New York served 531 per thousand, and Vermont served 163 per thousand of this group. The next highest service jurisdiction was the District of Columbia, which served 148 per thousand of this group, followed by Massachusetts, which served 139 per thousand, New Hampshire, serving 117 per thousand, and Wisconsin, which served 108 per thousand of the target group (see Figure 4). At the lower end of this scale, almost no home health service needs were met through Medicaid. Arizona, which does not have a Medicaid program, of course, satisfied no claims for Medicaid home health

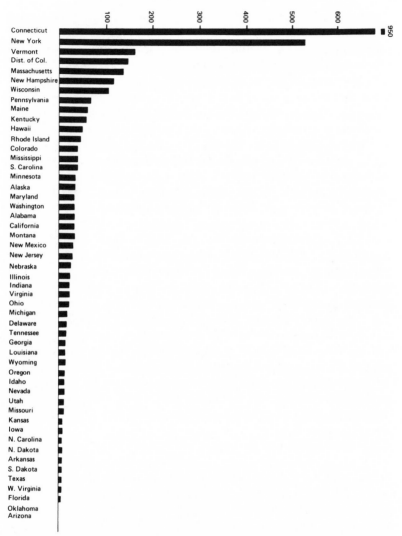

FIGURE 4. Number of Recipients of Home Health Services under Medicaid per 1,000 Disabled Elderly, FY 1977.

services *under this program.* However, Oklahoma, which does have a program, also satisfied almost no claims under the Medicaid program. Florida satisfied the service claims of only 4 per thousand of disabled elderly. Arkansas, South Dakota, and West Virginia served 6 per thousand, while Iowa, North Carolina, North Dakota, and

Texas served 7 per thousand of this population under the Medicaid home health program.

Thus, in terms of meeting needs under this program, a few states made considerable use of the program; many made almost no use at all. *Most* states made only negligible use of home health services under Medicaid.

Using a somewhat grosser measure, the inequity of funding distribution becomes dramatic. *Slightly over 81.2 percent ($145.7 million) of total benefits expended in fiscal 1977 ($179.5 million) under the Medicaid home—health service provisions were provided by New York State.* New York State residents constituted 8.7 percent of the nation's chronically ill elderly. The next highest state in terms of proportion of Medicaid benefits provided under the home health service titles was Maryland (3.8 percent) (U.S. Department of Health, Education, and Welfare, Health Care Financing Administration, 1979: 50-51). Another way to look at this problem is by considering the Medicaid home health dollars spent per disabled elderly in the states' populations (see Table 1). New York spent $386.91 per disabled elderly in the state. This is followed by the District of Columbia with $109.55, and Massachusetts ($55.02) and Vermont ($51.44). At the other extreme, Florida spent only $0.77 per disabled elderly, Iowa spent $1.48, and Missouri spent $1.79. Of the 44 states with Medicaid home health expenditures, the average expenditure per disabled elderly was $21.91. Such divergence of expenditure level indicates substantial within program inequities in terms of provision of home health care services.

Title XX—Social Security Act

Title XX of the Social Security Act is, as we have previously noted, the major program providing federal funds for the financing of social services. Certain of the service categories of Title XX are primarily, although not exclusively, focused on the elderly population.[6] Exact figures on elderly participation in Title XX programs are not tabulated nationally. This is due to failure to require such reporting in the federal statute and federal regulations. As with Medicaid, states have wide latitude and state's policies vary widely

---

[6]These services include day care and foster care for adults, home-delivered and congregate meals, home management, homemaker and chore services, protective services for adults, and group activity centers for the elderly.

TABLE I+

Dollars Expended Per Disabled Elderly for Home Health Services by Medicaid, FY1977

State*	Estimated # of Disabled Elderly (18% of elderly population)	Medicaid Expenditure for Home Health Services (in Millions)	Medicaid Expenditure for Home Health Services Per Disabled Elderly
New York	374,760	$ 145.7	$ 386.91
Dist. of Columbia	12,780	1.4	109.55
Massachusetts	123,660	6.8	55.02
Vermont	9,720	0.5	51.44
Kentucky	68,760	1.8	26.17
Maine	23,400	0.6	25.64
New Hampshire	16,740	0.4	23.89
Hawaii	11,340	0.2	17.64
New Jersey	145,440	2.4	16.50
Minnesota	81,720	1.3	15.91
Alabama	71,640	1.1	15.35
Montana	14,220	0.2	14.06
Indiana	99,720	1.2	12.03
Washington	69,480	0.8	11.51
New Mexico	17,640	0.2	11.34
S. Carolina	44,460	0.5	11.25
Nevada	9,180	0.1	10.89
Delaware	9,540	0.1	10.48
Virginia	81,720	0.8	9.79
Rhode Island	21,240	0.2	9.42
Nebraska	35,820	0.3	8.38
Connecticut	61,200	0.5	8.17
Maryland	64,620	0.5	7.74
Colorado	40,320	0.3	7.44
N. Carolina	95,400	0.7	7.34
Pennsylvania	257,760	1.8	6.98
Idaho	15,120	0.1	6.61
Illinois	214,920	1.4	6.51
Wisconsin	96,120	0.6	6.24
Louisiana	65,340	0.4	6.12
Georgia	82,080	0.5	6.09
Michigan	153,000	0.9	5.88
Utah	17,640	0.1	5.67
Tennessee	83,700	0.4	4.78
California	393,300	1.8	4.58
Ohio	199,800	0.9	4.50
Mississippi	47,880	0.2	4.18
Texas	221,040	0.7	3.17
Oregon	49,320	0.1	2.30
Arkansas	51,300	0.1	1.95
Kansas	52,740	0.1	1.90
Missouri	111,960	0.2	1.79
Iowa	67,320	0.1	1.48
Florida	259,920	0.2	0.77

+ U.S. Department of Health, Education, and Welfare, Health Care Financing Administration, Data on the Medicaid Program: Eligibility, Services, Expenditures, 1979 Edition, Baltimore, Maryland, 1979, pp. 46–47; U.S. Department of Health, Education, and Welfare, Health Care Financing Administration, Medicaid State Tables, Fiscal Year, 1977, Baltimore, Maryland, 1980, unpublished preliminary data.

* The following states show no expenditures for home health services in FY 1977: Alaska, Arizona, North Dakota, Oklahoma, South Dakota, West Virginia, and Wyoming.

in the determination of eligibility for Title XX in-home services.[7]

While all Title XX funded programs are not designed for the disabled or functionally limited elderly, homemaker services are clearly targeted to this group. Our analysis is based on this assumption. While we do not know how many recipients of homemaker services are elderly, SSI recipients make up 62 percent of those receiving homemaker services.

[7]Because annual utilization figures were not available for 1977, our analysis of the Title XX program is based on quarterly figures.

There were six states that did not provide homemaker services through Title XX (Alaska, Arkansas, Indiana, Utah, Vermont, and Wisconsin). In addition, seven states had programs which were so small as to be negligible (Connecticut, Florida, Hawaii, Illinois, Kentucky, Oklahoma, and Oregon). Even the states with the largest programs served less than 20 percent of the elderly disabled population (see Figure 5). California serves 196 per thousand; Montana,

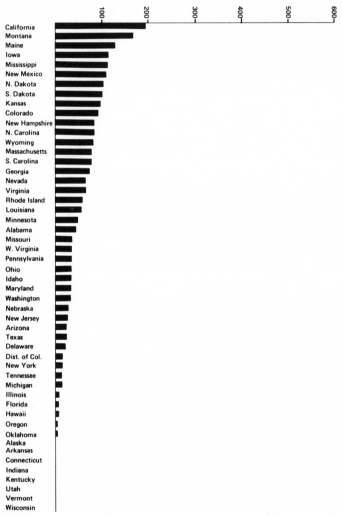

FIGURE 5. Number of Recipients of Homemaker Services under Title XX per 1,000 Disabled Elderly, Oct.-Dec. 1977.

170; Maine, 129; Iowa, 114; Mississippi, 112; New Mexico, 111; North Dakota, 107; and South Dakota, 102. The rest served less than 10 percent, with the average of 45 states serving only 56 per 1,000 disabled elderly. Thus clear inequities in the distribution of in-home services are evident in the Title XX program. Title XX is not a good vehicle for providing equitable state-by-state benefits which meet the social service needs of the chronically ill elderly.

TITLE III—THE OLDER AMERICANS ACT

Under the Older Americans Act, social services funding is divided into two categories: (1) access services and (2) in-home services. *Access services* costs are considered to be those costs incurred for activities which bring services to people or bring people to services: transportation, outreach, information and referral. *In-home services* costs are considered to be those costs which are incurred for delivery of services to an elderly person in his or her residence, and which are designed to assist the person receiving the service to continue to live independently *excluding* home delivery of meals which is covered under Title III, Part C, Subpart 2. In-home services include costs for homemaker and home health aides, visiting and telephone reassurance, and chore maintenance.[8] Our analysis will examine home health services and homemaker services (U.S. Department of Health, Education, and Welfare, Administration on Aging, undated a and undated b). When combining these categories, it appears that Mississippi served 149 per thousand of the targeted group; other states which made substantial use of this program were Colorado (143 per 1,000), New Jersey (131 per 1,000), Louisiana (125 per 1,000), and Hawaii (111 per 1,000)[9] (see Figure 6). At the other end of the scale, a number of states made no use at all of the Older Americans Act in fiscal 1977 in the categories indicated. These states were Alaska, Delaware, Idaho, Maryland, New Mexico, New York, North Carolina, North Dakota, Oregon, Rhode Island, and Wisconsin.

---

[8]In fiscal year 1980, local services for the aging were supported administratively by 610 area agencies on aging.

[9]The State of Montana shows an extremely high rate of usage of such funds meeting 95.5 percent of targeted need in 1977; however, when compared with its expenditure pattern it becomes apparent that Montana's figures are not reliable and that they appear to be due to reporting errors.

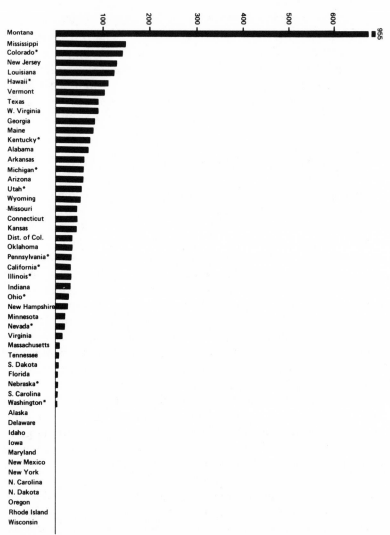

*FY 1977 data are not available. FY 1979 data has been substituted.

FIGURE 6. Number of Recipients of Home Health and Homemaker Services under Title III (OAA) per 1,000 Disabled Elderly, FY 1977.

The top five states in terms of utilization received over 20 percent of services; however, only 7.2 percent of the targeted chronically ill elderly resided in these states. The state-by-state inequity in use of funds is apparent here. The states which made no use of Older Americans Act service funds in the category of home health and homemaker services for the elderly constituted states with over 20 percent of the elderly disabled population in the United States. Service levels of 0 *clearly* indicate state-by-state inequity, as well as being inadequate in terms of meeting the needs of the target group.

In terms of examining expenditures for fiscal year 1977, we utilize the category of in-home services. This title is more encompassing than home health and homemaker services. However, the two largest items in this category are the two aforementioned titles. In fiscal 1977, 35 percent of federal Older Americans Act funds for in-home services were spent by New York State and 30 percent of such funds were expended by Pennsylvania. *Thus, 65 percent of the available revenues for in-home services under the Older Americans Act were expended by two states. When Connecticut's 7 percent expenditure is added we find that 72 percent of such service funds were expended by three of the fifty states (plus D.C.). According to our base figures, these states accounted for 16 percent of the disabled elderly population.*

The data which we have reviewed indicate the failure of the four federal programs to relate in-home health and social service funding to the needs of the chronically ill elderly on an equitable state-by-state basis. The patchwork nature of state-by-state funding results in gross inequities in utilization of funds and in levels of in-home services available to the disabled elderly.

INTERPROGRAM ADEQUACY AND A FURTHER EQUITY CONSIDERATION

Discussion of Methodology

In our analysis thus far, we have examined equity by comparing population served and expenditures in various states for each of the four federal programs which fund in-home services. We now turn to a discussion of program adequacy. In this analysis, we need to recognize that services from several of these programs are available in all states, with most states providing in-home services for the disabled elderly from all four funding sources. Thus the question of adequacy necessitates an examination of the total range of programs available in each state.

Of the programs we have examined, Medicare, Medicaid, and Title III provide home health services. All four programs provide personal care, and Title III and Title XX provide homemaker service. In our analysis of the adequacy of in-home service, we will add the number of recipients of service per thousand disabled in each state for each of the four in-home service programs as a measure of level of service provided (see Table 2). However, some reservations are necessary.

The sum of recipients from the four programs as an indicator must be considered cautiously for several reasons. First, many people may be double or even triple counted. For example, a person may use home health service under his/her Medicare benefit. When he/she reaches the limit of visits, the person may "spend down" and become eligible under Medicaid. The same person may receive homemaker service under Title III or Title XX. Another example of this problem would be program-shifting, due to the fact that the three programs utilizing both state and federal funds (Medicaid, Title XX, and Title III) do not have the same formula for federal-state matching. While Medicaid in some states provides federal matching at a 50-50 rate, Title XX required only 25 percent be provided by the state with the remaining 75 percent being funded by the federal government. As of FY 1982, Title XX requires no state match of federal funds. Thus, these states may find it advantageous to transfer home care patients from Medicaid-funded services to those services funded by Title XX (Trager, 1980: 30-32). Therefore, the numbers we have calculated have to be seen as maximums. Also, as previously mentioned, except in the instance of Title III, not all recipients of home health or homemaker service are elderly. They may be young, disabled adults, or children of abusive or ill parents. Thus again, the figures we are using are *higher* than the actual number of disabled elderly using the services.

Another caution regarding estimation of the adequacy of levels of service is the fact that being a recipient of service does not mean that the amount of service received was truly adequate to the need. While one individual might receive weekly homemaker services for an entire year, another might receive only one or two visits. Both would be considered to be receiving service, and count equally toward adequacy of service. Figures on number of visits by types of

TABLE II

Number of Recipients of Home Health and Homemaker Services
Per 1,000 Disabled Elderly, 1977, under 4 Government Programs[1]

State	# Elderly Disabled	Medicare[2]	Medicaid[3]	Title XX[4]	Title III[5]	Total
Montana	14,220	155	31	170	955[+]	1311
Connecticut	61,200	272	850	0	44	1166
New York	374,760	167	531	14	0	712
Vermont	9,720	412	163	0	103	678
Mississippi	47,880	263	39	112	149	563
Maine	23,400	286	61	129	80	556
New Hampshire	16,740	280	117	86	27	510
Massachusetts	123,660	250	139	80	9	478
Colorado	40,320	171	40	92	143**	446
Dist. of Columbia	12,780	243	148	15	36	442
California	393,300	166	31	196	32**	420
New Jersey	145,440	222	29	29	131	411
Pennsylvania	257,760	257	69	36	35	397
Louisiana	65,340	188	16	56	125	385
Rhode Island	21,240	259	46	60	0	365
New Mexico	17,640	187	30	111	0	328
Hawaii	11,340	150	51	8	111**	320
Alabama	71,640	163	31	44	70	308
South Carolina	44,460	166	39	80	2	287
Missouri	111,960	186	11	38	46	281
Wyoming	6,300	127	14	82	53	276
Georgia	82,080	89	16	76	82	263
West Virginia	39,420	119	6	37	89	251
Kentucky	68,760	116	59	0	72**	247
Texas	221,040	126	7	24	89	246
Wisconsin	96,120	136	108	0	0	244
Ohio	199,800	153	21	35	29**	238
Michigan	153,000	142	19	13	59**	233
Idaho	15,120	185	12	34	0	231
Maryland	64,620	162	33	33	0	228
Delaware	9,540	189	18	20	0	227
Florida	259,920	207	4	8	4	223
North Carolina	95,400	129	7	86	0	222
Kansas	52,740	61	8	100	43	212
Washington	69,480	145	32	31	2**	210
Illinois	214,920	141	22	9	31**	203
Arizona	45,000	120	0	24	58	202
Nevada	9,180	98	12	66	21**	197
Tennessee	83,700	154	18	14	7	193
Iowa	67,320	68	7	114	0	189
Minnesota	81,720	80	36	49	22	187
Virginia	81,720	82	22	66	13	183
South Dakota	15,840	57	6	102	6	171
Utah	17,640	102	12	0	56	170
Oregon	49,320	140	13	6	0	159
Nebraska	35,820	95	26	30	4**	155
North Dakota	13,860	36	7	107	0	150
Indiana	99,720	67	22	0	30	119
Arkansas	51,300	53	6	0	60	119
Alaska	1,620	62	34[+]	0	0	96
Oklahoma	62,820	56	0[+]	2	36	94

Total ($\bar{X}$) 4,229,640 (total)   56[5]

TABLE II (Continued)

*This figure is calculated as 18% of the elderly in the state in 1977--AOA figures.

[1]Figures for Title XIX and Title III are for the 1977 fiscal year; figures for Title XX are for the last quarter of the 1977 calendar year; Medicare figures are for the 1977 calendar year.

[2]U.S. Department of Health, Education, and Welfare, Health Care Financing Administration, "Medicare: Use of Home Health Services, 1977," Health Care Financing Notes, Baltimore, Maryland.

[3]U.S. Department of Health, Education, and Welfare, Health Care Financing Administration, Medicaid State Tables, Fiscal Year 1977, Baltimore Maryland, 1980, unpublished preliminary data.

(see footnotes next page)

TABLE II (Continued)

(4) Department of Health, Education, and Welfare, Office of Human Development Services, Social Services USA, First Quarter Report, FY 1978, Washington, D.C., Aug. 17, 1979. The figures for the Title XX Homemaker Program cited here are quarterly rather than annual figures. These figures are 4th quarter 1977 calendar year figures.

(5) U.S. Department of Health, Education, and Welfare, Administration on Aging, Title III Social Services Under Area Plans, Fiscal Year 1977.

**As 1977 figures were not available for these states, 1979 figures were used instead.

†Rounds to less than one.

(5) Based on 45 states with Title XX homemaker programs.

††This figure is suspicious as it is so much higher than other states. It is probably the result of an error in reporting.

staff provided rather than a mere head-count are needed in order to see how services are spread. Available data on expenditures per recipient show a wide variation by states and programs. Thus again, the numbers we are using show only that a certain number of persons received services and not that the level of service was indeed adequate to the need.

Also, we have been using the figure of 18 percent of the elderly population as an estimated "target population." However, when we begin to estimate need for in-home services, our target will be different from that of the number of disabled elderly. Many of the disabled elderly live with relatives, and these relatives may meet most or all of their care needs. Only 30 percent of the disabled elderly live alone, and many of these have family or other help living nearby. Unfortunately, we do not have available data to make an accurate estimate of level of need for services among the disabled elderly. However, there have been some studies of this population which may give us a rough idea of how many of these use in-home services beyond what they are receiving from informal or family supports (Applebaum, Seidle, and Austin, 1980; Gross-Andrew and Zimmer, 1978).[10] *Based on a review of these studies, we have made the assumption that only about 50 percent of the disabled elderly population would be likely to use home health care and other in-home services. Thus, the indicator of program adequacy utilized is provision of service at this 50 percent level. Also, if benefit levels*

[10]One weakness of these studies is that they measured need in a population at one point in time. Since level of need met is compared for service programs which operate over a 12 month period, a measure taken at a single point will underestimate annual need. Over a year's period, some persons who needed services will no longer need them, and some who did not will develop a need. An adequate service program would serve both groups. Thus, the number of recipients of an adequate program would be larger than the number in need at any one point in time.

*are found to vary as to adequacy on an interprogram basis, this
funding constitutes a further indication of interprogram inequity
with respect to provision of service relative to need across the four
programs under discussion.*

In the estimate of the overall adequacy of four combined federal
programs which follows, we will be using measures of utilization
which over-estimate the number of elderly disabled users and
estimates of need which under-estimate the need. It must also be
remembered that the figures from the different programs are not
totally comparable. While Medicare utilizes calendar year figures,
Medicaid and Title III present fiscal year utilization figures, and the
figures from Title XX program are quarterly figures. Also, with the
exception of Medicaid and Medicare figures, it often appears that
the states use different systems to compute usage. Thus the data in
the following analysis regarding adequacy of in-home service programs are subject to the qualifications noted.

Having reviewed the limitations of our data, we are proceeding
with our analysis. In so doing, we accept Gunnar Myrdal's conten-
tion that "it is better to paint with a brush of unknown thickness than
to leave the canvass blank" (Myrdal, 1972:71-72). We acknowledge a clear need for a national reporting system in these programs
so that consistent and reliable data can be obtained.

Findings

In our earlier analysis of equity in in-home service programs for
the disabled elderly, we have shown that many states make little or
no use of available programs. In these cases, inadequacy of service
can be assumed. Also, programs, such as Medicaid, which require a
"pauper's oath" to be sworn prior to gaining eligibility, limit the
adequacy of the benefits provided by eliminating from service
eligibility persons in need.[11]

In order to examine adequacy we sum the number of recipients
per thousand disabled elderly of four combined federal programs
which provide home health and homemaker services for the disabled
elderly (see Table 2). As we have noted, this section of the analysis
utilizes an estimate that 50 percent of the disabled elderly population
will be in need of such service. This means that to reach adequacy, a

---

[11]Of course such definitions are often based on state fiscal considerations rather than on
considerations for meeting the needs of low-income chronically ill elderly persons.

state should provide service to at least 500 per 1,000 disabled elderly in the state. *Our results show that even using figures which overestimate the numbers of recipients, only six states provided service at this level (see earlier note on Montana's Title III program).* These are Connecticut, New York, Vermont, Mississippi, Maine, and New Hampshire. With the exception of Mississippi, these are all Northeastern states. Connecticut and New York have large Medicaid home health programs; Vermont has an extremely large Medicare home health program. Mississippi and Maine fund in-home services largely through Medicare, Title XX, and Title III. New Hampshire has the same size Medicare program, but has more Medicaid home health services and fewer Title III or Title XX services.

Aside from these six states, the data show a rapid fall-off from the 500 per 1,000 disabled elderly level of need. Only 4 states (Massachusetts, Colorado, California, and New Jersey) and the District of Columbia, served 400-500 per 1,000 disabled elderly. Only 6 states served 300-400 per 1,000 disabled elderly. Fully 19 states served only 200-300 per 1,000 disabled elderly, and 12 states served less than 200 per 1,000!

If we look at the size of the elderly population in these states, given the assumptions of our analysis, we find that 12.5 percent of the elderly disabled lived in states where levels of home health and homemaker services were adequate, 16.3 percent lived in areas which were close to adequate (400-500 per 1,000), the remaining 71.2 percent lived in states where provision of this type of service was inadequate. Thus even when we summed across programs, over-estimating service provided and under-estimating need, we found that only a few primarily Northeastern states provided adequate service. Also, the data provide further evidence that even on an interprogram basis inequity exists in that a large majority of states do not provide home health and other in-home benefits to meet existing needs.

CONCLUSION

On the basis of our four-program study, we conclude that publicly supported home health and other in-home services for the chronically limited elderly in many states and regions were inadequate in that they often failed to meet the *national* needs of the chronically limited elderly on an interprogram basis. Neither was horizontal equity achieved under these programs—either separately, within each of the four stated programs on a state-by-state basis, or on an interprogram state-by-state basis. The failure to provide horizontal equity was less severe in the federally administered Medicare program. However, as this program is primarily a vendor payment system, adequacy of provision was most apparent where an extensive health delivery system had developed (certain urban areas) and less apparent in the absence of such development. Also, the Medicare program focuses on acute illness, rather than the chronic disease problems more commonly found in the elderly population. This program is also limited in that it is targeted toward medically sanctioned needs, rather than social needs also prominent in the chronically limited elderly population.

The other three programs discussed, Title XX of the Social Security Act, Title III of the Older Americans Act, and Title XIX of the Social Security Act (Medicaid) are all primarily state-run programs *without* specific federal requirements of the states with regard to fulfillment of particular goals related to providing community-based supports for the chronially ill elderly (U.S. Congress, House of Representatives, 1974; U.S. Health, Education, and Welfare, Health Care Financing administration, 1979; 50-51; Health, Education, and Welfare, Administration on Aging, 1979:1). For instance, Title XX of the Social Service Amendments of 1974 only provides appropriations to encourage ''. . . each State, as far as practicable under the conditions of that State, to furnish services directed at . . .'' broadly defined goals. Under Title III-A of the Older Americans Act, no federal service delivery goals for meeting the needs of the community-based chronically ill elderly are defined for State Agencies on Aging or Area Agencies on Aging. Indeed, the social service capacity of the program is admittedly a ''gap-filling'' one. Also, while home health care services for individuals 21 or older is a federally mandated Medicaid service upon the states for those states receiving federally supported financial assistance, one state, Arizona, lacks a Medicaid program, and one state, New York, received over 80 percent of federal program funds under the program. Clearly, the level of state provision of home health services under this program is not monitored by the national government. Moreover, such aid is only available on the basis of submission to a financial means test and not on the basis of functional need.

Thus, in addition to the observed failures of adequacy and equity of provision, we would note in the three programs of a federal-state nature, a clear failure by the national government to establish service delivery goals regarding adequate service levels for community-based assistance for the chronically ill elderly. In other words, such programs fail to establish a clear criteria with respect to public accountability for the state use of federal funds (Trager, 1980:31).

It is possible, even probable, that the overlap of all four programs does provide an adequate infrastructure of home health care and related social services for the chronically ill elderly *in some communities, and in some states.* However, it is clear that serious inequities exist and that the level of in-home services available is inadequate for the large majority of our disabled elderly population.

A need exists to establish a community-based system of health and social service supports which would enable many of the chronically ill elderly to maintain a position in the community in close proximity to caring relatives and friends. Such a family and community-oriented policy should be established by the federal government on the basis of systematically developed norms which would assure that this policy was adequate in meeting needs, equitably provided for all those in need of services, and which would establish clear national goals and public accountability for the use of federal funds to fulfill such goals.

REFERENCES

Applebaum, Robert A.; Seidl, Frederick W.; and Austin, Carol D. "The Wisconsin Community Care Organization: Preliminary Findings from the Milwaukee Experiment." *The Gerontologist,* 20 (June 1980), 350-355.

Burns, Eveline M. "Social Security in Evolution Towards What?" *Social Service Review,* 39 (June 1965), 129-140.

Callahan, Wayne. "Utilization of Home Health Services, 1977." *Medicare Program Statistics Report.* U.S. Department of Health, Education, and Welfare, Health Care Financing Administration, July 1979, unpaginated.

Davidson, Stephen N. "The Status of Aid to the Medically Needy." *Social Service Review,* 53 (March 1979), 97-105.

Gross-Andrew, Susannah; and Zimmer, Anna H. "Incentives to Families Caring for Disabled Elderly: Research and Demonstration Project to Strengthen the Natural Supports System." *Journal of Gerontological Social Work,* 1 (Winter 1978), 119-133.

Myrdal, Gunnar. *Asian Drama: An Inquiry Into The Poverty of Nations.* New York: Random House, 1972.

Nagi, Saad Z. "An Epidemiology of Adult Disability in the United States." Columbus, Ohio, Mershon Center, 1975 (mimeographed).

Ozawa, Martha N. "Individual Equity vs. Social Adequacy in Federal Old Age Insurance." *Social Service Review,* 48 (March 1974), 24-38.

Ozawa, Martha N. "Who Receives Subsidies Through Social Security, and How Much?" *Social Work,* 27 (March 1982), 129-134.

Ozawa, Martha N. "Issues in Welfare Reform." *Social Service Review,* ⁵
37-55.

Palley, Marian L. and Palley, Howard A. "A Call for a National Welfare
can Behavioral Scientist, 15 (May/June 1972), 681-695.

Palley, Marian L. and Palley, Howard A. "National Income and Servic
United States," in Dorothy B. James (ed.) *Analyzing Poverty Policy.* L
D.C. Heath, 1975, 241-252.

Palley, Marian L.; Palley, Howard A.; and Harkins, Daniel F. "The Nee
Income and Services Policy." *Policy Studies Journal,* 2 (Spring 1974)

Pfeiffer, Eric. *Multi-Dimensional Functional Assessment: the OARS Metho.*
Durham, North Carolina: Duke Center for the Study of Aging and Hum.
1976.

U.S. Congress, House. "Social Service Amendments of 1974," H.R. 93-1(
2nd Sess., December 19, 1974.

U.S. Congress, Senate, Special Committee on Aging. *Developments in Agir*
A Report of the Special Committee on Aging, 97th Cong., 2nd Sess., Fe

U.S. Department of Health, Education, and Welfare, Administration or
Report Fiscal Year 1978. Washington, D.C., 1979.

U.S. Department of Health, Education, and Welfare, Administration on ,
Status Report, Title III, FY 1977. Washington, D.C., undated a.

U.S. Department of Health, Education, and Welfare, Administration on ,
Status Report, Title III, FY 1979. Washington, D.C., undated b.

U.S. Department of Health, Education, and Welfare, Health Care Financ
tion. *Data on the Medicaid Program: Eligibility, Services, Expenditure*
Baltimore, Maryland, 1979.

U.S. Department of Health, Education, and Welfare, Health Care Financing
"Medicaid State Tables, Fiscal Year 1977." Baltimore, Maryland, 19
preliminary data.

U.S. Department of Health, Education, and Welfare, Health Care Financing
"Medicare: Use of Home Health Services, 1977." *Health Care F*
Baltimore, Maryland, undated a.

U.S. Department of Health, Education, and Welfare, Health Care Financing
Health Insurance, 1976: Summary Aged, undated b. (Xeroxed and unp

SECTION III

IN-HOME SERVICES
AND THE COMMUNITY-BASED
NETWORK OF SERVICES:
THE STATUS OF CURRENT
PROGRAMS AND A REVIEW
AND CRITIQUE
OF LEGISLATIVE PROPOSALS

Chapter 6

Selected Aspects of the Community Long-Term Care Package: Home-Based Care and Other Community-Based Services

In-home services should be viewed as the linchpin of a network of community-based services aimed at keeping the frail elderly and other disabled persons in an at-home setting where such a setting is appropriate. The purpose for writing this chapter is to attempt to sketch a picture of some significant dimensions of the infrastructure of community-based long-term care services in the United States with regard to availability, accessibility, and appropriateness of services. In attempting to draw this picture we were handicapped by the limitations of available data and the idiosyncratic nature of the available data with regard to completeness and incompleteness. Given these constraints, we have tended to focus on a discussion of some highly publicized community care projects, home health care and social care services, the state of adult day care services, and respite care. We will discuss national policy in support of housing for the elderly—as adequate housing is an essential prerequisite for community-based and in-home long-term care services. A summary discussion of congregate housing, congregate meals, and home meals as well as boarding homes and adult foster care is also included.

Our inquiry has faced us with an awareness that before national needs can be determined with regard to the extent of community-based and in-home long-term care for the elderly, we must develop a national commitment with regard to collection of necessary data and a census of available resources must be undertaken. It is with much concern that we note the lack of national commitment to undertake this task at the present moment. Our conclusion is that it is a task which very much needs to be undertaken.

COMMUNITY-BASED CARE

A substantial number of persons over age 65 could benefit from some form of community-based care. It has been estimated that some five million aged persons, aged 65 and over, who are living outside of nursing homes are limited in their ability to work, keep home, and undertake other major activities (U.S. Congress, House, Select Committee on Aging, 1980b:56). Robert and Rosalie Kane suggest that the choice between nursing home care and more community-centered care for the frail elderly should be viewed as alternatives in a continuum of care rather than dichotomies of service. Indeed they note that:

> The utility of alternatives often depends on the presence of a high quality, institutionally-based service capable of diagnostic and rehabilitative functions, temporary admissions for social reasons (e.g., vacations of caretakers) and high quality of services for that subset whose social and health needs might be better met in institutions. (Kane and Kane, 1980:252)

Thus, in Great Britain, geriatric hospital service is utilized to assess new admissions. Utilizing a triage system, patients deemed fit for rehabilitation for community living are routed to appropriate treatment centers and subsequently are reintegrated in the community. Similar systems apply in the Scandinavian countries. A few such experiments on a voluntary basis have been established in the United States. Such "geriatric centers" are primarily built around a long-term nursing home care facility (Expansion Committee, 1980). The Jewish Community Federation of Metropolitan New Jersey supports such a project in West Orange, New Jersey. This program is known as the Daughters of Israel Pleasant Valley Home Geriatric Center. In addition to a nursing home, the Geriatric Center operates a *day center* for the frail elderly which provides a daytime only program of medical, nursing, social, vocational, and recreational services to the frail, at-risk elderly; it also operates *Harel*—a program of congregate living for the elderly—in which the participants live in the community but share in the operating of their apartment with supervision and assistance provided by the staff of the Daughters of Israel Pleasant Valley Home. Also provided is a *Community Nutrition Program* targeted for elderly persons who are either unmotivated or unable to prepare meals. In this program, the Home prepares and delivers hot, nutritionally balanced kosher meals to several Senior Citizen Centers. Also *Digs,* a housing corporation, has been created by the Home in conjunction with the Jewish Community Federation. The Corporation operates 134 units of housing for the elderly in West Orange designed for the frail elderly and other handicapped individuals. The housing complex offers a congregate service package including one meal a day, and housekeeping and recreational program services. This congregate housing project is subsidized by the U.S. Department of Housing and Urban Development. The non-institutional services noted are viewed as part of a "continuum of care" for the elderly. In addition to such services, elderly persons are provided with consultation and diagnostic services, and medical care in the community. In addition, the Geriatric Center conducts educational programs for the medical community and the general public in the management of problems of the aging. It conducts training programs for geriatricians—nurses, social workers, nutritionists, psychologists, etc.—in conjunction with medical schools and universities, and finally, it will conduct research on problems associated with the aging of humans.

The variety of community services which are support alternatives to long-term care in nursing homes are outlined in the following chart (see Figure 1). Such services in the home include medical services, nursing services, health aids, personal care services, homemaker and chore services, and help with meals and transportation. Congregate services may be provided for those needy individuals in their own homes or in congregate housing facilities. Such congregate services may include congregate day care, meals, and social and recreational services. Other alternatives to long-term care in a nursing home include domiciliary care and adult foster care.

Community care services for the elderly are provided by a complicated network of federal funding sources (see Figure 2). Such programs are funded in part by federal agencies as diverse as the Health Care Financing Administration, the Office of Human Development Services, the Social Security Administration, the Administration on Aging, the Veterans Administration, and the Department of Housing and Urban Development. Prior to a discussion of some of the specific programmatic components of community-based, long-term care, it is necessary to note the complexity and the fragmentation of the current network of services.

COMMUNITY CARE PROJECTS

There are a number of dimensions to community-based care for the frail elderly, and potentially for other disabled individuals who could benefit by community care services. These are noted in the following description of the activities of the Wisconsin Community Care Project and the Triage Project of Connecticut.

Figure 1: Support Alternatives to Long-Term Care in Nursing Homes

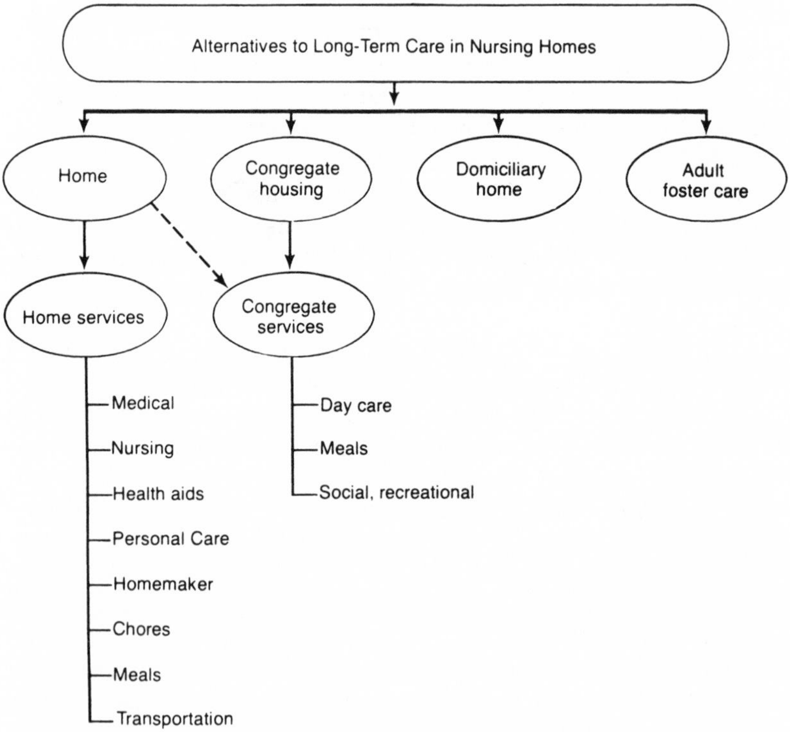

Source: Meyer Katzper. Modeling of Long Term Care (Washington, D.C.": Department of Health and Human Services, 1981), p.15.

Figure 2.: **Major Federal Programs Funding Community Services for the Elderly**

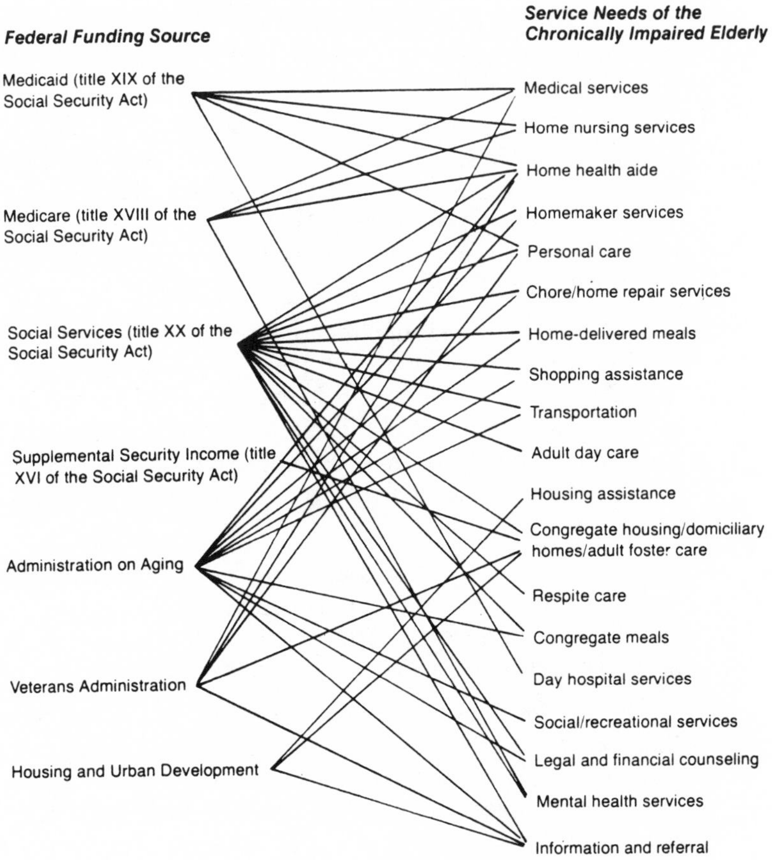

Federal Funding Source

Service Needs of the Chronically Impaired Elderly

Source: Meyer Katzper. Modeling of Long Term Care (Washington, D.C.: Department of Health and Human Services, 1981), p. 16

The Wisconsin Community Care Project includes a broad range of services to the disabled elderly population in the cities of LaCrosse and Milwaukee, as well as Barron County (Wisconsin). Such major services are (U.S. Department of Health, Education, and Welfare, Health Care Financing Administration, 1980):

— Skilled health care services . . . designed to prevent and relieve problems caused by physical and mental disabilities. Services include medical, surgical, and skilled nursing home care; immunization; prescribing and administering of medications; and health care instruction. Care is provided by appropriate professionals.

— Home health services include assistance with personal care, hygiene, prescribed exercises, medication, and incidental household services, such as meal preparation, shopping, and light housekeeping. Services are performed by home health aides, homemaker, and other qualified persons according to an established plan of care.

— Medical equipment and supplies are furnished to: (a) compensate for physical disabilities that interfere with a participant's independent functioning; (b) cosmetically correct a physical deformity; and (c) assist the nurse or her aide in providing necessary services. Care may be provided by an orthopedist, prosthetist, brace fitter, corsetierre, or other qualified personnel.

— Therapeutic medical services are provided in a rehabilitation center, or a hospital outpatient department. Physical services are usually performed by certified physical, speech, and occupational therapists, audiologists, and their trained aides.

— Home care/homemaker services assist the participant with day-to-day tasks in the home. Services may include any combination of laundry, shopping, transportation, housekeeping, personal care, meal preparation, financial management, errands, and companionship. The care may be provided by a member of the participant's family, a private home care provider, a homemaker aide, a homemaker, or other supervised paraprofessionals.

— Chore services consist of performing household tasks such as shopping, lawn mowing, snow shoveling, and minor painting.

— Home repair and reconditioning services cover such tasks as roofing, electrical and plumbing repair, and installation of wheelchair ramps, stairways, handrails, and grab bars. These services are performed by a handyman or a skilled craftsman.

— Meal services consist of the regular delivery of meals to the participant.

— Transportation services enable participants to travel to and from other services, and bring materials to them.

— Counseling services are designed to promote a sense of well-being within the participant by improving his ability to cope with stress. This includes treatment for mental, emotional, and social problems.

— Protective services are intended to protect participants who are vulnerable to abuse or exploitation.

— Legal and financial services cover such matters as taxes, contract disputes, medical assistance eligibility, court appearances, and resolution of complaints.

— Social therapeutic services and adult day care services offer supervised, planned programs which may include opportunities for companionship and self-education. These services are provided outside the participant's home by a social worker, or a qualified professional, or trained aides.

— Visiting services consist of regular visits to the participant's home for social contact and are generally performed by a volunteer.

— Companion services provide care and protection for the participant within his home on a day, night, or live-in basis.

— Housing services are provided for the participant on a short-term, long-term, or emergency basis. This includes finding new housing, and renovating existing housing.

Thus an imposing array of services has been included under the rubric of the community care services. While managed centrally, many such services were provided by contract. For example, the Milwaukee CCO concluded 40 provider contracts with 14 different services. Also, services such as homemaker/home health aide, transportation, and home delivered meals which had not been ordinarily provided under Medicaid showed a high rate of utilization.

Also, CCO clients had monthly medical assistance costs substantially below that of matched control clients, $197.87 as compared to $325.42. CCO clients utilized an average of 2.95 days of hospital care, as compared to control clients who utilized an average of 14.26 days of hospital care. Nursing home utilization also was lower for CCO clients—who averaged eight and one-half fewer days in nursing homes than the control group. The 1980 *Final Evaluation Report* of this project concluded that in spite of a higher cost of administration, the project ". . . was on the edge of cost effectiveness when compared to the regular Medical Assistance program . . . and had come close to adding a potentially important component to the continuum of care without additional cost to the Medical Assistance Program."

A similar array of services is also observed in the following description of Triage. Triage is a research and demonstration project supported by a grant from the Health Care Financing Administration (HCFA) which provided health care and social services to the elderly in a seven town area of Connecticut. It provided a single entry point for elderly persons to an extensive array of services. Also provided was a comprehensive assessment of health, social, financial, and environmental needs of the older adult which was "conducted by an inter-disciplinary team made up of a masters degree nurse clinician and a masters degree social service coordinator." Services were designed "to strengthen and support family and environmental support systems, rather than to replace them" (U.S. Congress, House, Select Committee on Aging, 1980c:12). Triage services included traditional Medicare services plus other waivered services allowed by HCFA in connection with the research and demonstration project.

The "Medicare" services were:

— Hospital,
— Skilled nursing facility,
— Physician,
— Outpatient services,
— Diagnostic services,
— Podiatry,
— Ambulance,
— Visiting nurse,
— Home health aide,
— Physical therapy,
— Occupational therapy,
— Speech pathology, and
— Durable medical equipment.

The "Waivered" services were:

— Intermediate care facility,

— Dental care,
— Dentures,
— Optical care,
— Eyeglasses,
— Audiological services,
— Hearing aids,
— Mental health counseling,
— Homemaker,
— Chore services,
— Companion,
— Prescription drugs and over-the-counter medication,
— Meals-on-wheels
— Ambulance (for non-emergency),
— Chaircar,
— Taxi service,
— Friendly visiting, and
— Legal services (U.S. Congress, House, Select Committee on Aging, 1980c:13).

The waivers also eliminated all coinsurance and deductible requirements, the then prevailing 3-day prior hospitalization requirement for skilled nursing facility placements, and the then prevailing limits on Medicare home health benefits. Such limits were:

> visit limitations of 100 days per illness period under Part A and 100 days per calendar year under part B; that patients be hospitalized for 3 days for eligibility under Part A; that the patient be homebound; and that a physician establish the plan of care. (U.S. Congress, House, Select Committee on Aging, 1980c: 13)

Of these limitations only the latter two still remain.

The population served by Triage was a frail elderly group, predominantly widowed females living alone—with limited financial resources and limited education. Upon initial assessment, 72.4 percent of the Triage group had heart and circulatory problems, and 22 percent had digestive problems. Many had more than one problem. Sixty-six percent had difficulty with tasks such as shopping, taking care of their financing and their medications, whereby they could maintain themselves independently. Eighty percent had good cognitive functioning—that is, they were able to relate to time, place, and location. Eighty-three percent did not have difficulty with feeding, bathing, or dressing themselves (U.S. Congress, House, Select Committee on Aging, 1980c:17).

In F.Y. 1978, among the 1747 clients who were served, Triage prevented or delayed 81,275 days of long-term institutional care (see Table 1). This situation was estimated to result in a financial savings of $1,688,329. Triage was able to prevent institutionalization in nursing homes of 20 to 30 percent of its clients through the utilization of alternative care, ambulatory care, and home care. Forty-eight percent of the clients had improved or maintained their ability to carry out basic community living activities.

In reviewing the Wisconsin Community Care Project and the Triage Project, we have tried to present a view of the myriad activities which are part of community care for the aged. We also have noted some of the social and economic benefits associated with such care.

A recent Congressional report includes a discussion of Triage, the Wisconsin Community Care Organization Program (CCO), as well as four other experimental efforts in long-term health care for the elderly. Except for Triage (which is primarily linked to Medicare), all of these programs are primarily linked to Medicaid as a point of departure for determining client eligibility for new and revised community-based services, or by using Medicaid supported services as core services under the projects. Most of the projects take advantage of various provisions under the Social Security Act that allow experimental waivers of the general statutory requirements that service be statewide, that allow services to be introduced which are not ordinarily part of the State's Medicaid plan, and that allow modification of existing eligibility criteria.

In addition to the programs already mentioned, other projects reported on included the Georgia Alternative Health Services Project (AHS), the Monroe County (New York) Assessment for Com-

Table 1

Institutional Days Saved - Fiscal Year 1978

Prevented admissions	61,320
Delayed admissions	19,955
Total	81,275

Source: U.S. Congress, House, Select Committee on Aging.
          Long Term Care for the 1980's, 1980, p. 13.

munity Services Project (ACCESS), the Virginia Nursing Home Pre-Admission Screening Program, and the State of Washington Community Based Care Systems for the Functionally Disabled Program (CBC). A primary target group of such programs is the frail elderly.

Such programs generally expanded client eligibility and service availability criteria. With respect to client eligibility, one site in the Wisconsin CCO program provided services for individuals whose incomes exceeded the State's Medicaid Program eligibility criteria; New York's ACCESS Project made available assessment services for all county residents *18 years of age or older* regardless of income status; and Washington's CBC system included a number of Title XX eligible persons in its program. Non-income related criteria used as determinants of eligibility for the project include such factors as:

Individuals "at-risk" of institutionalization within a certain time period, e.g., three months, six months; individuals living in the community who have been referred for institutional care, or who are "in crises" and in imminent danger of institutionalization and who have disabilities which interfere with successful home-based functioning; individuals at the point of discharge from a hospital or nursing home; institutionalized non-Medicaid eligible individuals judged at risk of converting to Medicaid eligibility status due to depletion of income and resources; and/or institutionalized individuals for whom institutional care is determined inappropriate. (U.S. Congress, House, Committee on Energy and Commerce, 1981: 6-7)

The various projects developed differing need assessment criteria. Such criteria were multi-dimensional, relating to such factors as: degree of independence in performing activities of daily living, health status, current living arrangements, and the availability of social and environmental supports.

Except for the Virginia Nursing Home Pre-Admission Screening Program, which provided for no addition to the supply of existing services and emphasized a screening process, all projects combined existing community-based services with new or modified services under Medicaid or Medicare waiver authority. Services not otherwise available except through such expanded waiver authority included in the Monroe County ACCESS Program: "For Medicaid eligible clients: limited housing improvement; home maintenance/chore services, temporary financial assistance for housing, rental, transportation; friendly visiting; moving assistance; and respite care for family members" (U.S. Congress, House, Committee on Energy and Commerce, 1981:8). The respite care could involve temporary institutional or non-institutional care for ACCESS clients being cared for by family members or other individuals in an informal support network. The Washington CBC program utilized such additional "waivered" services as personal care, mini-bus transportation, and adult day care. The waiver mechanism enabled most projects to provide a significant number of complementary community-based health and social services to clients with similar needs through a central funding source, as well as the ability to compensate for services which were not otherwise available.

It is unclear that such community-based care will reduce nursing home costs—due to the continued high demand for nursing home care. Nevertheless, such community-based services have been found to constitute a less costly alternative either for clients whose release from hospitals has been delayed until they are more self-sufficient, or for nursing home care, which often is not the most appropriate alternative. Where appropriate, such services are preferred by many frail elderly and may result in improved functioning for the home-based frail elderly (U.S. Congress, House, Committee on Energy and Commerce, 1981:6-7).

HOME CARE

In examining the development of home care programs in the United States, it is important to determine the extent of, and the need for, such home-based services (Dunlop, 1980; Pegels, 1980; Doherty, Segal, and Hicks, 1978).[1] According to the National Home Caring Council, more than 5,000 agencies in the United States now provide both homemaker and home health aide services—categories combining health and social services (National HomeCaring Council, 1981). A more complete source limited to information with respect to home health care is Medicare certification data for home

---

[1]The Congressional Budget Office estimated that in 1976, 20 to 40 percent of all institutionalized persons were inappropriately placed and could be in less intensive settings where adequate community-based care was available. See U.S. Congressional Budget Office, 1977: x.

health care agencies available from the Health Care Financing Administration (U.S. Department of Health and Human Services, Health Care Financing Administration, 1981). As of September 30, 1981, there were 3,136 home health care agencies certified by the Medicare program. Of these, 1,231 were governmental—operated by state, county, and municipal health departments, 544 were private non-profit services operating outside hospital auspices; and 436 were hospital-based non-profit programs. Five hundred fifteen were run by the Visiting Nurse Association. Two hundred ninety-seven were proprietary services. Fifty-four were partly governmentally funded, non-profit sponsored programs, and fifty-nine were categorized as "all others."[2] A 1980 change in federal law allows proprietary plans to be federally certified by Medicare without state licensure. Federal authorities expect this change to result in a substantial increase in federal certification of proprietary home health care plans under Medicare.

More encompassing than home health care, many of the frail elderly have a need for the services of a home care system. According to Moore, home care implies a complex of services including the "services of health professionals; homemaker services; and home maintenance and repair service" (Moore, 1981:57). The notion of home health aide services has been federally specified as services involving "personal care and certain limited household services which include changing the bed, light cleaning, food shopping, and help in cooking." Homemaker services have been defined as: home management (cooking, cleaning, laundry, and related tasks); personal care (assistance in bathing, dressing, eating, walking, skin care, etc.); supportive activities (tasks outside the home such as shopping); and health care management services (such as accompanying the patient to health care services and working with others during a home health visit) (U.S. Department of Health, Education, and Welfare, National Center for Health Services Research, 1979: 4). Home care thus involves both health services, functional maintenance services as well as social services. Federal funding for such services is provided in the manner indicated by Table 2.

A recent General Accounting Office study documents some gaps

---

[2]Such home health agencies vary both in availability to meet regional needs and in the number of services provided. Among services provided by Medicare-certified home health care agencies are nursing care, physical therapy, speech therapy, medical/social services, home health aide services, intern and resident services, nutritional guidance, pharmaceutical services, appliances and equipment, and vocational guidance. Many such home health agencies provide only nursing care and one or two other services.

Table 2

COMPARISON OF ESSENTIAL CHARACTERISTICS

OF FOUR PROGRAMS FUNDING IN-HOME SERVICES

	Social Security Act			Older Americans Act
	Title XVIII	Title XIX	Title XX	Title III
Services authorized:				
Nursing	yes	yes	no	yes
Therapy	yes	yes	no	yes
Home health aide	yes	yes	yes	yes
Homemaker	no	no	yes	yes
Chore	no	no	yes	yes
Medical supplies and appliances	yes	yes	no	no
Program eligibility requirements:				
Client must meet age requirement	yes	no	no	yes
Client must meet income requirement	no	yes	yes	no
Client must need part-time or intermittent skilled nursing care	yes	no	no	no
Client must be homebound	yes	no	no	no
Services to client must be authorized by a physician in accordance with a plan of care	yes	yes	no	no
Services must be included in State Plan	(a)	yes	yes	yes
Administration	Federal	State	State	State
Funding	open ended	open ended	capped	capped

a/ Federally administered program--no State Plan required.

Source: U.S. General Accounting Office. Improved Knowledge Base Would Be Helpful In Reaching Policy Decisions On Providing Long-Term, In-Home Services For The Elderly. Washington, D.C., October, 1981, p. 26.

in community home care services. It notes that between 10 and 22 percent of persons 65 years of age and older are not receiving all the homemaker/chore and personal care services that they need. Of those elderly whose needs are being met, 76 percent of the cost of these services are provided by family and friends (U.S. General Accounting Office, 1981). Thus, often public programs are not being utilized to reach patients in need of such home care services.

The goals of an adequate community home care service might be stated as follows (Moore, 1981:63):

1. Coordinated health and social services focused on the home.
2. Federal resources to stimulate an expanded and better coordinated system enabling providers of services to deliver an adequate scope, range, and duration of services for home care consumers.
3. Health and social service resources better balanced between home, ambulatory, and institutional care.
4. An appropriate mix of professional, paraprofessional, and volunteer services.
5. A holistic view of services by staff and board levels of provider agencies so that the services of various agencies are coordinated and gaps in services are both recognized and met.
6. A focus on quality of care.

ADULT DAY CARE

Another part of the long-term care services package is adult day care. In 1971 federal support was provided for a few experimental adult day care programs. By 1978 over 600 programs had been developed serving about 13,500 persons (U.S. Congress, House, Select Committee on Aging, 1980a:52). By 1980 over 800 programs were in operation.

A "1980 Adult Day Care Survey" conducted by the Subcommittee on Health and Long-Term Care of the House Select Committee on Aging indicates that the most frequently provided service of state-funded day care programs was nutrition (89 percent). This was followed by social services (86 percent), health services (75 percent), and transportation (71 percent) (U.S. Congress, House, Select Committee on Aging, 1980a:52).

In 1981, Medicaid supported 47 adult day care programs in Massachusetts, 23 in New York, and 13 in California (U.S. Congress, House, Select Committee on Aging, 1980a:52). Georgia had 10 such programs; the State of Washington had 9; New Jersey had 8; Kansas and Maryland had 6 and 2, respectively. Under Title XX of the Social Security Act in 1981, 40 states supported 297 adult day care programs. The leader in this area was Alabama with 38 programs. Other states maintaining between 10 and 20 Title XX supported programs included North Carolina, Texas, New Jersey, Illinois, Mississippi, Tennessee, Ohio, Maryland, and Pennsylvania. Other sources of funding for adult day care services include Title III of the Older Americans Act, philanthropic sources, revenue sharing, and the United Way.

The 1980 U.S. Adult Day Care Directory classifies adult day care programs in terms of three modes. These are as follow (U.S. Congress, House, Select Committee on Aging, 1980a:23):

> *Restorative programs* are those offering intensive individual care plans for each participant. Where prescribed, therapeutic services are provided on a one-to-one basis by certified specialists with constant health monitoring and provision of a therapeutic activities program.

> *Maintenance programs* are those with the capability (in terms of health professionals on the staff and appropriate equipment) to carry out a care plan for each participant based on recommendations from the personal physician (or clinic) and developed by the multidisciplinary program team. Services provided include health monitoring; supervised therapeutic, individual, and/or group activities and psychosocial services.

> *Social programs* show wide variations in nature and scope. Some social programs place great stress on health maintenance, with nursing services an integral part of the total program; other social programs create formal linkages with local clinics or health departments and transport participants to needed services; still other programs are concerned solely with socialization and lunches.

While day care programs offer a variety of different health, social, and supportive services, the following services are offered in different combinations according to the type and availability of funding, the community resources, and the needs of participants (see Table 3).

Although day care programs are characterized as medical, social,

Table 3:   The Adult Day Care Services Package

Basic services offered by most programs:

- general nursing
- social work
- recreation activities
- assistance with activities
  of daily living

- supervision of personal hygiene
- lunch
- referral to community agencies

Additional services frequently offered:

- two meals a day
- snacks
- nutritional counseling
- meals-on-wheels
- medical doctor care
- speech, physical, and occupational therapy
- psychiatric
- psychological

- diagnostic
- rehabilitative nursing
- music therapy
- reality therapy
- health education
- sheltered workshop
- laundry
- transportation
- home care

Source: "Adult Day Care: An Overview," National Institute of Senior Centers' (NISC) Senior Center Report, a newsletter published by the National Council on the Aging, Inc. 1 (August/September 1978), 4.

or psycho-social in focus, most programs are really a blend of health, social, and psycho-social services. Table 4 provides a brief overview of service objectives and types of clients.

While adult day care serves a variety of disabilities which are not limited to an elderly clientele, the frail elderly are a primary target group. The "1980 Adult Day Care Survey" found that the dominant funding source for adult day care was Title XX, followed by Medicaid.[3] It concluded that: "In a time of an increasingly elderly population, high costs of nursing home and ICF [Intermediate Care Facility] care, it appears that day care is functioning as a needed alternative on the local level . . ." (U.S. Congress, House, Select Committee on Aging, 1980a:154).

RESPITE CARE

Adult day care programs may include a dimension of respite care for family caregivers. Often the primary caregiver of the elderly husband is his wife. A 1973 study of Lopata found that 46 percent of

[3]Claims have been made for the cost-effectiveness of adult day care vis-à-vis nursing home care. In terms of per diem governmental program costs of alternative care in California, Ellen Stein Harris reported that one adult day care program saved the government of that state $182.57 per month, or $2,202.81 per year (Harris, 1976).

Table 4: Adult Day Care Programs*

Type of Service	Major Service Objective	Type of Client
Medical Service	To provide health care resources to chronically impaired individuals.	Individual has chronic physical illness or disabilities; condition does not require daily medical intervention but does need nursing and other health supports.
Psycho-social Services	To provide a protective or transitional environment that assists the individual in dealing with multiple problems of daily coping.	Individual has history of a psychiatric disorder; could reactivate and/or suffer from mental deterioration (organic or functional) that places him in danger if not closely supervised.
Social Services	To provide appropriate socialization services.	Individual's social functioning has regressed to the point where, without formal, organized social stimuli, overall capacity for independent functioning would not be possible.

Source: "Adult Day Care: An Overview," National Institute of Senior Centers' (NISC) Senior Center Report, a newsletter published by the National Council on the Aging, Inc. 1 (August/September 1978), 4.

*Adapted from Philip G. Weiler and Eloise Rathbone-McCuan. Adult Day Care: Community Work with the Elderly (New York: Springer Publishing Co., 1978).

the widows in the study had cared for their husbands at home before their deaths. Forty percent of them had cared for their husbands for more than one year (Lopata, 1973; Crossman, London, and Barry, 1981:464). This is not a surprising finding since women tend to be younger than their husbands at marriage and tend to live longer than their husbands (Shanas, 1979).

The Marin Senior Day Services (Mill Valley, California) respite care program is a model program which provides an example of the support services often needed by wives or other relative-caregivers of the chronically limited elderly. In this instance the program was viewed as a program supporting the wives of chronically limited elderly males. The problem necessitating respite care is noted in the report of Crossman et al.:

Adult day care is available 4 days a week and the majority of wives take advantage of this respite. Day care did not, however, obviate the need for home care. For many of the wives, the task of getting the husband ready to go to the day center is sometimes more than the hours of respite are worth and some can manage only 1 or 2 days a week for this. In other cases, the husband is too disabled to tolerate a full day of activity or is totally bed ridden. Furthermore the day care program does not provide such personal care services the husbands require such as bathing. Few of the women could afford the rates charged by the community's proprietary for-profit home care agencies on a long term basis and no agency offered services on a sliding fee scale. All of the couples are just above the eligibility level for publicly subsidized services and whatever savings the couple does have, the wives are struggling to retain. Knowing that they will probably outlive their husbands, they fear the prospect of an impoverished existence. This is also one of the factors in their reluctance to institutionalize the husband since the high cost of nursing care would rapidly deplete their limited assets and, in effect, pauperize the wife in the process. (1981:467)

The Marin Senior Day Services Project in 1979 developed a respite project with two major service components: (1) home care and (2) overnight respite care. The home care service component provided one full-time nurse whose time was divided among 10 to 15 wives who requested service (Crossman, London, and Barry, 1981:468). Such services were gradually limited to 4 hours a week per couple. When coupled with day care it expanded the respite available to women while providing needed assistance in the home. For those husbands not requiring personal care, the nurse provided companionship and supervision while the wife dealt with errands and appointments. Such home care was provided without charge. In addition to such services, the home care nurse had detected undiagnosed hypertension among both patients and caregivers. The nurse also found that she was called upon to teach about the causes and effects of chronic diseases in explaining a husband's behavior or functional problems. In addition to assisting in household tasks, such as shopping and meal preparation, the nurse provided emotional support for the wives.

With regard to overnight respite, Marin Senior Day Services developed a licensed six-bed adult group residential facility. The program of care ran from Thursday morning to Monday morning.

Wives reserved space in advance for their husbands. Respite care might be provided from 24 hours to a full 4 days. The facility was staffed by nurses who were affiliated either with the respite care project or the day care program.

As the Crossman report notes, for elderly couples who participated it was an "opportunity to have periods away from the intense interaction and stresses inherent in their relationship" (Crossman, London, and Barry, 1981:469). It was particularly a respite for the wives—all of whom had not had a vacation in many years. Whether institutional or in the home, respite care provides needed psychological and physical support for participants in the "natural support system."

PUBLIC SUPPORT OF HOUSING FOR THE ELDERLY [4]

Over 20 percent of all U.S. households in 1982 were headed by persons 65 years of age or older. A number of federal housing programs pay particular concern to the problems of elderly renters and home owners (see Table 5).

The Section 202 direct loan program provides for construction of specially designated low income housing for elderly and handicapped persons. Since its enactment in 1974, it has produced 79,000 units occupied by elderly persons. In addition, the Department of Housing and Urban Development (HUD) was authorized in 1978 to award grants to public housing authorities and Section 202 sponsors in order to provide meals and supportive services to partially impaired elderly and handicapped persons which would allow them to remain in their own dwellings and keep them out of institutionalized settings.

More general programs focusing on the needs of low income renters also heavily serve older Americans. The "existing housing section" of the Section 8 program, which provides rental assistance for households occupying existing units, and the "new construction/ substantially rehabilitated portion" of the Section 8 program are aimed at increasing the supply of affordable housing to low income persons eligible for rental assistance. In 1981, 50 percent of the 1.9 million units constructed under these programs were occupied by persons 65 years of age or older.

---

[4]U.S. Congress, Senate, Special Committee on Aging, 1982:212-221.

It is in order to indicate how the programs we have mentioned operate. Under the Section 8 program, HUD enters into assistance contracts with owners of existing housing or with developers of new or substantially rehabilitated housing. Under such contracts, a specified number of units will be leased by households meeting federal eligibility criteria. Payments by the federal government paid to owners and developers under such assistance contracts make up the difference between what the rental household can afford to pay for rent and what HUD has determined is the "fair market rent" of the unit. As of June 1981, HUD estimated that about 597,000, or 37 percent, of a total of over 1.5 million Section 8 units were occupied by elderly persons; over 283,000 (or 54 percent) of newly constructed units were occupied by such older persons. Prior to fiscal year 1982, assisted families made rental payments which amounted to not less than 15 percent nor more than 25 percent of their net income. Under the Omnibus Reconciliation Act of 1981, the tenant share was increased from not more than 25 to not more than 30 percent of net income. For existing tenants of Section 8 units, upward adjustments in rent were to be made gradually over a five year period.

The Section 202 program has been the primary federal financing instrument for the construction of housing for older Americans in order to enable them to maintain their self-sufficiency and independence. Such projects generally operate as other Section 8 housing with the additional stipulation that such housing be specifically designed to meet the needs of the frail elderly and handicapped persons. For fiscal year 1982, appropriations were provided for the development of 17,200 such units.

A final housing program which deserves mention is public housing. This program is the oldest federal program providing housing for the elderly. Over 45 percent of its more than 1.2 million units are occupied by the elderly. It is a federally financed program established by the United States Housing Act of 1937, and operated by local non-profit public housing agencies (PHAs). Such PHAs generally own the local projects. They may issue notes and bonds to finance acquisition, construction, and improvement of projects. Federal financial assistance is primarily in the form of annual contributions to underwrite the PHA debt service. Congress also has provided some subsidy for tenant rents, particularly as such rents have not kept pace with increased operating expenses. Since 1971, PHAs have had the authority to use federal revenues for the provi-

Table 5

SUMMARY OF HUD HOUSING UNITS FOR THE ELDERLY

(All figures represent number of projects/units currently insured by FHA unless otherwise noted.)

Section No.: Program: Status	Projects	Units	Value	Approximate elder units	Percent of elders	Cumulative figures through—
CONSTRUCTION PROJECTS						
Title II: Low-income public housing: Active.	10,750	1,200,000	(9)	[1]552,000	46	Sept. 30, 1979
202: Direct loans for housing for elderly and handicapped:						
Inactive[2] ————	+330	45,275	574,580,000	45,275	100	1977.
Active[3] ————	1,006	90,323	4,130,154,957	79,185	89	June 30, 1981.
	495	66,285	1,158,117,347	66,285	100	Do.
231: Mortgage insurance for housing for elderly: Active.	3,532	355,101	5,718,508,463	21,918	7	Do.
221(d)(3): Multi-family rental: Active.	5,239	582,313	13,908,371,752	75,745	13	Do.
221(d)(4): Housing for low- and moderate-income families: Active.						
235: Home ownership assistance for low- and moderate-income families:						
Inactive[2]————	7472,059	473,032	8,456,660,790	(9)	(9)	Program revised.
Active ————	78,034	78,134	2,768,814,179	————		June 30, 1981.
207: Multifamily rental housing: Active.	2,633	275,588	3,944,141,865	3,380	1.2	Do.
236: Rental and co-op assistance for low- and moderate-income families: Inactive.	4,056	435,231	7,492,815,583	55,784	13	Do.
202/236: 202/236 conversions: Inactive.	181	8 28,059	480,098,460	[8]28,059	100	Do.
232: Nursing home and intermediate care facilities: Active.	1,300	147,336	1,676,509,129	147,336	100	Do.

Table 5, cont'd

SUMMARY OF HUD HOUSING UNITS FOR THE ELDERLY

Section No.: Program: Status	Projects	Units	Value	Approximate elder units	Percent of elders	Cumulative figures through --
NONCONSTRUCTION PROGRAMS						
84: Low-income rental assistance:						
Existing:[4] Active ----	10,990	916,704	(9)	265,492	28	Do.
New construction:[4,5] Active.	8,225	524,586	(9)	283,741	54	Do.
Substantial rehabilitation:[4,5] Active.	1,654	117,904	(9)	41,394	35	Do.
312: Rehabilitation loans: Active.[6]	86,004	(9)	(9)	6,243	7.25	Sept. 30, 1980.
23: Low rent leased housing: Inactive.[2]	(9)	163,267	(9)	54,000+	35	Approximately Dec., 1975.

1 Data do not indicate how many of these units are designed specifically for the elderly.
2 Figures for original program reported through program revision.
3 Figures for revised sec. 202/8 represent cumulative project reservations through June 30, 1981.
4 Figures represent cumulative fund reservations through reporting date.
5 Figures do not include sec. 8 commitments attached to sec. 202/8 fund reservations.
6 Figures represent loan commitments only.
7 Figures represent number of mortgages.
8 Beds.
9 Not available.

Source: U.S. Department of Housing and Urban Development, 1982.

sion of congregate dining facilities and equipment for such facilities in public housing projects. While little development of such congregate facilities has occurred, some of these services are provided in PHAs by local service agencies funded under the Older Americans Act, Medicaid, and/or Title XX. The Omnibus Reconciliation Act of 1981 requires public housing tenants to pay up to 30 percent of the household's adjusted income on rent (up from 25 percent), and new tenants must meet an eligibility test of 50 percent of the area median income. Federal funding was provided for the development of 30,396 new units of public housing in fiscal year 1981, and for 24,000 new units in fiscal year 1982.

CONGREGATE HOUSING AND MEALS, BOARDING HOMES AND ADULT FOSTER CARE

Other forms of community-based care include congregate housing and adult foster care. Initially, subsidization of congregate housing for the frail elderly was authorized under the Housing and Urban Development Act of 1970. Such authorization has been renewed by later amendments. A congregate housing situation "offers a minimum service package that includes some on-site meals served in a common dining room, congregate meals, plus one or more of such services as on-site medical/nursing services, personal care, or housekeeping" (Lawton, 1976:239).

In 1978 the Congregate Housing Services Act was passed (U.S. Congress, Senate, Special Committee on Aging, 1982:219-221). The Act authorized HUD to award specific grants to public housing authorities and Section 202 housing sponsors in order to provide nutritional meals and supportive services for partially impaired and handicapped residents which would allow such persons to remain in their own homes and out of nursing homes or other expensive institutions. A primary target group of such grants is the frail elderly. Such grants were to run from three to five years and they required supplemental funding from community sources to support delivery of the specified services. Local area offices on aging would coordinate existing local services with congregate housing services. Congregate housing services program (CHSP) projects were required to provide at least two meals a day, seven days a week, at centrally located dining facilities. Homemaker, housekeeping, personal assistance, counseling, transportation, as well as other needed supportive services could be provided under the program. Participants in the program were required to pay a fee for services received on the basis of their ability to pay.

By May 1981, 55 grants had awarded a sum of $16 million to various projects. By the end of 1981, most projects were operational and serving 2,200 elderly persons. Preliminary data indicate that such projects have helped individuals in the throes of a physical or mental crisis remain in their own dwellings; another trend indicates that a number of individuals have been released from institutional settings and placed in CHSP projects. The implication of the latter finding is that many such persons were unnecessarily placed in nursing homes because of the lack of available residential arrangements providing supportive services.

While this program was *not* renewed in 1982, Senator John Heinz (R., Pennsylvania) has noted the value of the projects in the following comment:

> Preliminary data collected by HUD and the American Association of Homes for the Aged . . . indicates that the program has been overwhelmingly successful in achieving its purposes. Premature institutionalization is being prevented . . . the development of housing for the partially impaired elderly and the handicapped is being stimulated . . . Federal health-related expenditures are being reduced . . . . (U.S. Congress, Senate, Special Committee on Aging, 1982:220-221)

Congregate meals also are encouraged by Title III of the Older Americans Act. The Title III nutritional programs have as their goal improving the health of program participants as well as seeking to attract isolated older persons to locations where needed services and social opportunities are present (U.S. Congress, Senate, Special Committee on Aging, 1982:405).

The Older Americans Act stipulates that congregate nutritional services be available at least once a day, five days a week. Such services are to be provided along with such needed support services as outreach, transportation, counseling, recreation, education, and information and referral. Many congregate meal locations have developed into senior centers serving a number of the needs of older Americans. Home delivered nutrition programs are based on a determination of need for service. Such meals must be served at least once a day to individuals who are homebound due to illness, incapacitating disability, or a severe transportation problem (U.S. Congress, Senate, Special Committee on Aging, 1982:405).

In fiscal year 1980, there were 1,185 nutrition agencies operating 12,556 congregate nutrition sites providing meals and support services in Administration on Aging supported programs (U.S. Congress, Senate, Special Committee on Aging, 1982:387). Over three million elderly persons received such nutrition services—62.5 percent of whom were low income elderly persons. More than 145 million meals were served under the program. About 15 percent of such meals were delivered to homes of persons who were unable to attend congregate sites because of long- or short-term impairments. The irregularity of meals received under the nutritional program was not sufficient to maintain a goal of nutritional adequacy through program meals, although they did serve as a focal point of community socialization for many elderly consumers.

Many infirm elderly also live in boarding homes which absorb the federal supplementary security income (SSI) payments of the residents. The State of New Jersey, which licenses 3,500 boarding homes housing many elderly persons, has indicated that to comply with current fire regulations owners would need 13 million dollars in loans (Hanley, 1981:B17). Congresswoman Maria Bragg (D., New York) commenting on boarding home fires which have killed large numbers of elderly residents notes:

> These boarding homes are federally subsidized infernos for the indigent. The indiscriminate dumping of older Americans from mental institutions and nursing homes into facilities like boarding homes is a deepening national disgrace. (Hanley, 1981:B1)

Clearly, this form of shelter is not a currently desirable part of community-based long-term care for the frail elderly.

Another form of sheltered housing is adult foster care. It is foster care "for persons in need of care and protection in a substitute family setting for a planned period of time" (Newman and Sherman, 1977:436). Funding for such programs is largely reliant on Title XX social services funding; however, some monies are available through state departments of health and mental health programs, and in most cases the foster family is paid a percentage of the SSI or Social Security check of the recipient of foster care. Such programs are essentially state developed and administered. Consumers of this service are generally low income elderly without relatives and in need of family-surrogates to maintain a place in the community. These programs are similar to boarding home programs but they minimize the likelihood of abuse through (1) selection of acceptable homes; (2) limits on the number of patients; (3) placement service for clients, and (4) supervision of the foster home by social service staff. Many of these programs were established to serve former mental patients, but some serve frail elderly as well.

A recent development has been the extension of foster home programs for those frail elderly who are in need of skilled nursing care. There are a few prototype programs in the country. All were developed by hospitals with private funding. Two of these programs have successfully made the transition from grant funding to funding through the State Medicaid Program (Massachusetts General Hospital and the Johns Hopkins Hospital). In general, the Medical Assistance patient pays for about half of the cost through his/her SSI check. The State Medicaid Program pays the other half plus the administrative costs.

Program staff are primarily social workers and nurses, although some programs make use of nurses from existing home nursing services such as the Visiting Nurses Association (VNA). Staff recruits caregivers, evaluates home environments, provides training for caregivers, selects appropriate patients, matches agreeable patients and caregivers, and provides ongoing supervision and support for both patient and caregiver.

Only one of these programs has been carefully evaluated. The Johns Hopkins Community Care Program employed an experimental design in which the outcome of foster care was compared to nursing home care. While the final results are not yet available, preliminary analysis shows that:

1. Foster care patients are less disabled than is the entire nursing home population. This is because the least functional patients are screened out of community care because of excessive care needs.
2. Foster care patients are less likely than other patients to have family support. This is probably because when families decide not to provide care themselves, they are not comfortable with the idea of another family caring for their relative.
3. Foster care may be more acceptable to some ethnic racial groups than others. At Johns Hopkins, the program was more acceptable to Blacks both as caregivers and as patients.
4. The Foster Program was clearly less costly than was nursing

home care. The cost savings may be in the range of twenty to thirty percent.
5. After up to one year in the Program, the patients in the foster care homes were no worse off in physical and mental functioning than were the nursing home patients, and in some areas they may have been better off.

Foster home care programs appear to have the potential to provide care for a wide range of frail elderly. They have the advantage of being more flexible and providing more individualized care than do institutions. They are also clearly less expensive. However, there is the danger that unless careful supervision is provided, substandard care and even neglect and/or abuse will result.

Foster home programs may provide a viable alternative for those elderly who are without adequate family support and who are too disabled to be cared for in their own homes. However, at present, this alternative is not widely available. Nor is this availability likely unless Medical Assistance programs (as the largest source of nursing home funding) become convinced that the cost savings will not be offset by too great an expansion of the supported population.

CONCLUSION

Perhaps the linchpin of community services for the majority of the frail and disabled aged is personal support services. In their landmark study, *Social Services in International Perspective: The Emergence of the Sixth System,* Kamerman and Kahn note the importance of development of an infrastructure of community services for the aged with particular emphasis on what they refer to as social care services. Such services are defined as encompassing "that cluster of practical, helping measures such as homemaker-home-health, personal care and hygiene, delivered meals, shopping, chore, escort, reassurance, and visiting services." They also note that such services "include both in-home and out-of-home services, and they could be available to the aged living in ordinary housing as well as to those living in special or congregate housing; could encompass aspects of health care; and could include both long- and short-term care" (Kahn and Kamerman, 1980:303-304). Such care services should be readily available to those who need them without the presence of a financial barrier.

A community-based health and social care system would establish the right of the frail elderly to chose to live in the least restrictive environment. The availability of such services lessens the pressure for inappropriate referrals to institutional facilities such as nursing homes. Appropriate in-home services allow many frail elderly to maintain themselves in a non-institutional setting. In the case of those elderly who need extensive care, there should be alternatives to nursing home care. Families who chose to provide such care need the support of counseling, financial aid, day care (if appropriate), as well as institutionally based respite-care facilities. For those frail elderly who do not have this type of family support (a natural support system), foster home programs, adequately funded to provide close supervision and training, should be widely available.

REFERENCES

Brody, Elaine M. "Women's Changing Roles, The Aging Family and Long-Term Care of Older People." *National Journal* (November 27, 1979), 11-16.

Crossman, Linda; London, Cecilia; and Barry, Clemince. "Older Women Caring for Disabled Spouses: A Model for Supportive Services." *The Gerontologist,* 21 (October 1981), 464-469.

Doherty, Neil; Segal, Joan; and Hicks, Barbara. "Alternatives to Institutionalization for the Aged: Viability and Cost-Effectiveness: A Review of the Recent Literature." *Aged Care and Services Review,* 1 (January/February 1978), 2-16.

Dunlop, Burton D. "Expanded Home-Based Care for the Impaired Elderly: Solution or Pipe Dream?" *American Journal of Public Health,* 70 (May 1980), 514-519.

Expansion Committee, "Report of Sub-Committee on Geriatric Center—Daughters of Israel Pleasant Valley Home Geriatric Center," West Orange, New Jersey, November 3, 1980.

Hanley, Robert. "New Jersey Homes for Aged Draw Congressional Anger," *New York Times,* March 10, 1981, p. B17.

Harris, Ellen S. "Day Care for Senior Citizens." *Los Angeles Times,* October 3, 1979. (Reprint.)

Kane, Robert L. and Kane, Rosalie A. "Alternatives to Institutional Care of the Elderly: Beyond the Dichotomy." *The Gerontologist,* 20 (June 1980), 249-259.

Kahn, Alfred J. and Kamerman, Sheila B. *Social Services in International Perspective: The Emergency of the Sixth System,* New Brunswick, New Jersey: Transaction Books, 1980.

Lawton, M. Powell. "The Relative Impact of Congregate and Traditional Housing on Elderly Tenants." *The Gerontologist,* 16 (June 1976), 237-242.

Lopata, Helena Z. *Widowhood in an American City.* Cambridge, Mass.: Schenkman, 1973.

Moore, Florence. "Community Home-Care Services and Reallocating Health System Resources," in Robert Morris, ed., *Allocating Health Resources for the Aged and Disabled,* Lexington, Mass.: Lexington Books, 1981.

National HomeCaring Council. "News Release." New York, New York, September 1, 1981.

Newman, Evelyn C. and Sherman, Susan R. "A Survey of Caretakers in Adult Foster Homes." *The Gerontologist,* 32 (October 1977), 436-439.

Pegels, C. Carl. "Institutional vs. Non-Institutional Care for the Elderly." *Journal of Health Politics, Policy, and Law.* 5 (Summer 1980), 205-212.

Robins, Edith G. "Adult Day Care: Growing Fast But Still for Lucky Few." *Generations.* (Spring 1981), 22-23.

Shanas, Ethel. "The Family as a Support System in Old Age." *The Gerontologist,* 19 (April 1979), 169-174.

U.S. Congress, House, Committee on Energy and Commerce. *Experimental Efforts in Long-Term Health Care for the Elderly.* Report prepared for the Sub-Committee on Health, 97th Cong., 1st Sess., Washington, D.C., June 1981.

U.S. Congress, House, Select Committee on Aging. *Adult Day Care Programs,* Hearings before the Sub-Committee on Health and Long-Term Care, 96th Cong., 2nd Sess., April 23, 1980a.

U.S. Congress, House, Select Committee on Aging. *Families: Aging and Changing,* Hearings, 96th Cong., 2nd Sess., November 24, 1980b.

U.S. Congress, House, Select Committee on Aging. *Long-Term Care for the 1980's: Channeling Demonstrations and Other Initiatives,* Hearings before the Sub-Committee on Health and Long-Term Care, 96th Cong., 2nd Sess., February 27, 1980c.

U.S. Congress, Senate, Special Committee on Aging. *Development on Aging: 1981, Vol. 1,* A Report of the Special Committee on Aging, 97th Cong., 2nd Sess., February 22, 1982.

U.S. Congressional Budget Office. *Long-Term Care for the Elderly and the Disabled.* Washington, D.C.: U.S. Government Printing Office, February, 1977.

U.S. Department of Health, Education, and Welfare, National Center for Health Services Research. *Effects and Costs of Day Care and Homemaker Services for the Chronically Ill: A Randomized Experiment.* Washington, D.C., 1979.

U.S. Department of Health, Education, and Welfare, Health Care Financing Administration. "Report on Wisconsin Community Care Project." Washington, 1980. (Reprint.)

U.S. Department of Health and Human Services, Health Care Financing Administration, "Telephone Inquiry." Baltimore, Maryland, November 13, 1981.

U.S. General Accounting Office. *Improved Knowledge Base Would Be Helpful in Reaching Policy Decisions on Providing Long-Term, In-Home Services for the Elderly.* Washington, D.C., 1981.

Chapter 7

In-Home and Other Community-Based Long-Term Care: A Critical Review of Some Legislative Proposals and Recent National Legislation

This chapter addresses the public policy implications of our research findings. In this section, we will review critically two 1980 legislative proposals concerning in-home and other community-based services presented to the U.S. Congress, and the subsequent passage of relevant Congressional legislation. Additionally, a 1981 legislative proposal is discussed. We will examine these recent legislative trends and their potential strengths and weaknesses regarding the development of community-based in-home services, as well as community-based long-term care services which are often supportive of in-home care. As a postscript, we have examined the possible impact of "cut-back" funding on the development of in-home and other community-based care.

THE PACKWOOD BILL

Description

The most encompassing recent proposal for the development of community-based long-term care facilities was S.2809 (Non-Institutional Long-Term Care Services for the Elderly and Disabled). This bill was introduced in 1980 by Senator Robert Packwood, (R., Oregon) and would have created a Title XXI of the Social Security Act by combining all home health services under Medicare (Title

XVIII), Medicaid (Title XIX), and Social Services (Title XX).[1] The bill would have applied to such services as home health services, homemaker-home health aide services, adult day care, and respite care services. Such home health services would differ from Medicare in that skilled is dropped from the definition of nursing care, and the category home health aide services is replaced by the category homemaker-home health aide services. (Such services would include personal care such as bathing, exercising, personal grooming, assistance with getting in and out of bed, household care services such as light housekeeping, purchasing and preparation of food, and maintaining a safe living environment.) In addition, the bill provided for elimination of the 3-day prior hospitalization provision under Part A of Medicare (which subsequently has been eliminated) as well as the Title XVIII requirement that the individual receiving service be homebound.

Adult day care services would have been made available under the bill as would respite care services. Adult day care services were defined as regularly provided services to an individual in a multipurpose senior center, intermediate care facility, hospital rehabilitation center, or center or agency for the handicapped. Services, which were to be provided on a less than 24 hour per day basis, could have included: provision of meals, personal care, recreation and educational activities, physical and vocational rehabilitation, and health care services. Respite care services of up to 336 hours (42 days) per calendar year would have been provided. Such services were defined as temporary services for an individual who is unable to care for himself and is in need of service due to the absence of the usual care provider. The individual needing the caregiver would need to be dependent on the caretaker in order to receive such services.

Unlimited visits would have been provided for home health services, homemaker-home health aide services, and adult day care *except* that a copayment of 10 percent would have applied (to a maximum based on a percent of income) for visits in excess of 50 per

---

[1]A similar bill, S.861, was introduced into the 97th Congress by Senator Packwood and Senator William Bradley (D., New Jersey). The bill would have established Title XXI as a six-year demonstration concerned with acute and long-term care services for persons aged 65 and over and for chronically disabled persons. It makes provision for statewide demonstration projects which would have as their mandate to test the implementation of an organized system of non-institutional services for acute and long-term care patients. Three different methods of payment—fee schedules, prospective reimbursement, and capitation payments— would be tested under the proposed project.

calendar year. The bill also provided that reimbursement to providers be on the basis of a fee schedule for each service reflecting urban and rural differences and takes into account the full-time average direct wage cost per visit, the average transportation cost per visit, the indirect wage cost per visit, and an administrative cost allowance which would not exceed 20 percent of the total cost of a visit. Initially, the program would be introduced on a 3 year demonstration project basis with ten demonstration projects.

Screening, assessment, and establishment of a plan of care would be undertaken by Preadmission, Screening, and Assessment Teams (PATs). Such teams would function under the direction of a physician. Such teams would consist of a registered nurse, nurse practitioner, or physician assistant (in some instances); a social services worker; where necessary, a qualified professional in the field of mental retardation or developmental disabilities; where necessary, an occupational therapist; and a volunteer senior citizen advocate or a volunteer advocate for the disabled, whichever was appropriate. The functions of the PAT would be: to conduct a health status and functional assessment of each individual seeking Title XXI services, to develop a plan of care for persons deemed in need of service, to conduct a periodic reassessment of each person receiving service to find out if further services are required, to assist each person in obtaining services from appropriate providers, to keep the individual's personal physician aware of the individual's progress, and to conduct a health status and functional assessment for each individual entering a nursing home to insure appropriate placement.

Critical Assessment

In terms of the policy implications of our findings, a nationally administered program with statutory definitions regarding procedures and functions as envisioned in this bill would be a positive improvement over the current fragmented and uncoordinated nature of federal funding of home health care and other in-home services. In reference to current Title XVIII provisions regarding home health care services, the bill reflected an acceptance of the need for noninstitutional home health care on a long-term basis, and often unrelated to "cure" of an acute illness. The proposed dropping of the three day hospitalization requirement of Part A of Title XVIII represented a meaningful change over the then existing law in its recognition of the chronic, long-term nature of many of the physical

problems of the frail aged and the disabled. The expanded definition
of homemaker-home health aide, adult day services, and respite
care services would have provided a meaningful package of necessary services for those with chronic limitations who need some assistance in order to function in their communities and outside an institutional nursing home setting. Also, it offered an alternative of
community-based services which could replace overlong hospital
stays for recuperative patients. The bill also would have provided a
mechanism for avoiding the stigma and humiliation of requiring a
means test for receipt of services as is the case under Medicaid programs.

The suggested presence of copayment requirements for home
health services, homemaker-home health aide services, and adult
day care services after 50 visits in a calendar year might serve to
discourage those with chronic limitations and their caregivers in
need of such services from seeking them. The limitation of days for
respite care raises the problem of what one does if the service is
needed and the statutory 336 hours of service has been exceeded.
Also, while the bill would have allowed for a tax credit of $100 a
year for families caring for dependent elderly relatives to assist such
families to meet the rising costs of goods and services for caring for
such persons, the sum involved was insignificant. However, the
idea is good and a higher dollar limit could be set. Even more
desirable would be a system of government payment (or substantial
tax credits) for family members' home improvements and for provision of care by family members to the frail elderly and the disabled.
This approach has been successfully tried under some Medicaid programs. Another problem with the bill is the general Medicare vendor payment approach. The bill provides for payments; it does not
set up statewide or regional needs measures, nor does it provide
capital funding in sparse health service delivery areas; neither does
it have the authority to enforce a needed level of care. Thus, the bill
does little to overcome regional disparities regarding adequate
delivery of service; nor does it take sufficient measures to see that
high quality services are provided. The stipulation of the necessity
of a state plan requiring the meeting of certain levels of service and
the provision of supporting funding would have immeasurably
strengthened this proposal. Also, a statement that the combining of
home health and in-home service titles of Title XVIII, XIX, and XX
would not result in a lowering of current service levels would have
been in order. That is, states should be required to at least maintain

current levels of service regarding home health and other in-home services.

Another issue which was raised by this legislative proposal was that PAT must be under the general direction of a physician. While this title may have a rationale with respect to home health care, many in-home services are social care services and might be more appropriately directed by a social worker or a professional in the mental retardation or developmental disabilities areas. The language regarding PAT general direction could perhaps be tightened to state that where medical evaluation is a critical matter the PAT be under the direction of an appropriately specialized physician (gerontology or rehabilitative medicine); that in other cases other appropriately trained persons such as social workers or other specialists, with specialization in the area of gerontology or disability, direct the PAT.

THE WAXMAN BILL

Description

In 1980, another more limited bill seeking to expand community-based services was introduced in the Congress. This bill was an amendment to Title XIX (Comprehensive Assessment and Community Based Services, H.R. 6194) introduced by Congressman Henry Waxman (D., California).

The bill provided for comprehensive assessment and services for individuals likely to be in need of a long-term skilled nursing facility or intermediate care facility services. Individuals who were so assessed also would be assessed as to the feasibility of community-based long-term care alternatives to such institutional care. Community assessments were to consist of a direct personal assessment by trained individuals *of all factors:* including, among others, financial resources; medical, psychological, and social needs; architectural barriers and other environmental factors; family and community support; and the ability to live independently with appropriate in-home services. With respect to the service alternatives to institutional long-term care, the state medical assistance plan would need to provide such community-based long-term care services as: nursing services on a part-time or intermittent basis; home health aide services; medical supplies, equipment, and supplies suitable for the home; physical therapy, occupational therapy, and speech pathology and audiology services; adult day care services; respite care, short-term full-time nursing care, homemaker services, and nutritional counseling.

Under this plan, states providing services would require deliverers of service to meet professional standards (including state licensure), and generally to provide such services *without limitation as to amount, duration, and scope.* The state plan would establish minimum and maximum levels of reimbursement regarding types of care and services. Comprehensive assessments and services would receive federal funds either at a level of 25 percent above ordinary Medicaid levels or 90 percent, whichever was less. (That is, they would have ranged from 75 percent federal payment levels to 90 percent federal payment levels.)

Critical Analysis

On the positive side this bill recognized the complexity and the often largely social care nature of assessment for home health and other in-home care and simply provides that such assessment be provided by "trained individuals." It was positive in that a physician need not be the "directing" person for such assessment; it was negative in so far as there is a need for some further explication as to whom adequately fits the title "trained individual."

Another positive feature of this bill was its requirement of a state plan of service for eligibility for the high level of federal reimbursement involved. Such a plan cannot generally limit service to eligible individuals as to amount, duration, and scope—thus services under this title were to be comprehensive. In reality, however, services will only be as comprehensive as state reimbursement and facilities development policies require. Experience with Medicaid indicates that in a federal-state matching grant program with largely state administration, a great degree of variability will occur with regard to levels of service. This legislative proposal encouraged the states to utilize the long-term care alternative of community-based home health care and in-home services; it did not require the states to actually do so. As we have noted, it encouraged comprehensive care in the areas of home health care and other in-home services. On the basis of the prior experience of the Medicaid program, it is unlikely that a truly available, accessible, and comprehensive system of home health care services would have been implemented nationally under this title if it had been passed by Congress. With respect to another dimension of the bill, the language regarding state obligations for levels of service and quality of services was quite general and it remains to be seen as to whether future federal regulations or administrative oversight policies clarify the state's obligations with respect to levels of home health service and other in-home care services and quality control of such services. We believe it would be desirable to establish such national standards regarding state obligations for maintaining levels of service and insuring quality of services.

Subsequent Legislative Output

While the Packwood Bill did not pass Congress, it did trigger certain important Congressional modifications of Medicare in 1980. These Medicare Amendments eliminated the requirements under Part A of a prior three day stay in a hospital prior to eligibility for Part A home health services; it also eliminated the one hundred day limit on services under Part A and Part B and provided for unlimited days of service. However, such service remains limited by physician authorization that it is part of treatment for an acute illness. Furthermore, occupational therapy was added, in 1980, as an included primary home health care service, although it has since been eliminated as a primary service.

While the Waxman Bill did not pass, it triggered further congressional concern with provision of Medicaid-related in-home and community-based care as an alternative to nursing home care.

In the Omnibus Reconciliation Act of 1980, Congress provided for demonstration projects in no more than 12 states regarding the training and employment of welfare recipients as homemakers and home health aides "to elderly or disabled individuals, or other individuals in need of such services" where such services were not otherwise available and where the absence of such services could ". . . be increasingly anticipated as to require institutional care." Such authorized homemaker and home health aid services could include intermittent or part-time assistance with respect to "(A) personal care, such as bathing, grooming, and toilet care; (B) assisting patients having limited mobility; (C) feeding and diet assistance; (D) home management, housekeeping, and shopping; (E) health-oriented record keeping; (F) family planning services; and (G) simple procedures for identifying potential health problems." Federal reimbursement would be at a 90 percent federal level.

Under Section 2176 provisions of the Omnibus Reconciliation

Act of 1981, the Medical Assistance Program, upon request by a state and approval by the Secretary of Health and Human Services, may offer home and community-based services under a state-approved plan to eligible individuals ". . . pursuant to a written plan of care (for) individuals with respect to whom there has been a determination that but for the provision of such services to individuals would require the level of care provided in a skilled nursing facility or intermediate care facility the cost of which could be reimbursed under the State plan." Such Medicaid assistance would include case management services, homemaker/home health aide services, and personal care services, adult day health, habilitation services, respite care, and "such other services" requested by the State and approved by the Secretary of Health and Human Services. Such approval involves a waiver by the Secretary of Health and Human Services of Medicaid statutory requirements related to the specific types of services offered as well as the requirement that services be statewide.

The major significance of the Section 2176 provision of this legislation is the inclusion of a range of both health and personal care services, as well as the inclusion of a case management function.[2] Thus the law provided legislative recognition of the social, as well as the medical, requirements of community-based long-term care within the framework of the Medicaid program. This legislative enactment, while certainly important and desirable, contains no federal mandate for required provision of such services and, of course, ties provision of such services to a means test. It occurs within a framework of decreasing eligibility of needy individuals for such services due to the implementation of a federally mandated, more stringent means test than had previously applied.

THE HATCH BILL

Description

A Community Health Services Act (S.234), sponsored by Senator Orrin G. Hatch (R., Utah), has been introduced in the 97th Congress. It would allow for grants to public and non-profit private en-

---

[2]This case management function was defined as a system which placed responsibility for locating, coordinating, and monitoring a group of services with a specified person or institution.

tities for the specific purpose of meeting the initial cost of establishing and operating home health programs; in addition, loans would be available to proprietary home health care facilities for such purposes. Training grant money for homemaker/home health aide training programs also would be provided under the bill. This proposal positively recognizes the need to create an infrastructure of available services rather than merely providing a vendor payment system for clients. Where services are of poor quality or unavailable, the vendor payment system does little good for the client.

While not encompassing as broad a package of community-based services as the Packwood Bill, the Hatch Bill would include, as new *primary* services under Medicare, homemaker/home health aide, as well as occupational and respiratory therapy. Household care services would include food purchase and preparation, plus light housekeeping. (Transportation would be paid for in connection with covered home services.) Occupational and respiratory therapy would be reimbursed on a 100 percent basis, as would homemaker/ home health aide services received in connection with skilled nursing care, and physical or speech therapy. When offered without the aforementioned stipulated services, individuals qualifying for home health aide services, solely based on the need for such assistance, would be reimbursed at a 50 percent basis. Definitions regarding eligibility and benefits of home health services under Medicare also would be applicable under Medicaid.

Critical Analysis

Thus, the bill provides for broadened availability of enumerated community-based services. While intended as a device for seeing that only necessary homemaker/home health aide services are utilized, the 50 percent co-insurance requirement may discourage many needy elderly from obtaining such assistance.

The bill does provide for the treatment of chronic care as well as acute conditions under the Medicare program. It seeks to stimulate an increase in the number of providers by allowing the Secretary of Health and Human Services to waive the requirement that home health services be provided by a home health agency. Such utilization of a waiver process on the quality of care would require careful monitoring. Finally, the bill provides for a $500 refundable tax credit for taxpayers providing home care for a qualified dependent. This provision provides an admirable incentive for support of family members and others providing in-home care for the frail elderly and other disabled individuals.

The Hatch Bill, through its modest liberalization of benefits and its tax credit provision, would encourage the provision of appropriate community-based care for the frail elderly. Its loan and grant provisions constitute a recognition of the need for building an adequate and accessible infrastructure of available home health services. The provision of grants for the development of training programs for professional and paraprofessional personnel to provide home health services shows a desirable concern for the quality of delivery of home health services. In its scope it would constitute a desirable increment to the current status of publicly financed community care programs, and a step forward in establishing an adequate, accessible, and appropriate national infrastructure of home health and other in-home services.

THE IMPLICATION OF ECONOMIC CUTBACKS: A POST-SCRIPT

The Omnibus Budget Reconciliation Act of 1981 placed limits on the federal share of Medicaid. These limits call for reduction of federal matching payments to each state by 3 percent in fiscal year 1982, 4 percent in fiscal year 1983, and by 4.5 percent in fiscal year 1984. States could reduce the level of such limitations by such actions as adoption of a qualified hospital cost review program, recovering an amount equal to 1 percent of federal payments by controlling fraud or other program abuse, and by holding Medicaid spending increases below a certain target level. Federal matching payment reductions would be lowered where unemployment in the state was greater than 150 percent of the national average.

The impact of this legislation in a number of states has been the adoption of policies to limit Medicaid nursing home payments, and to place tighter restrictions on the transfer of assets by the elderly to relatives in order to gain eligibility. A number of states also have established preadmission and screening programs in order to limit ''less appropriate'' admissions to nursing homes. Such Medicaid cut-backs may not only limit the supply of nursing home care, but the limitation of available funds may prevent development of complementary community-based and in-home care on a statewide basis for the frail elderly and other individuals with significant disabilities.

Also, the Omnibus Reconciliation Act of 1981 cutback funding available for social services under Title XX of the Social Security Act. It authorized fiscal year 1982 spending at $2.4 billion—a 20 percent cut in such spending from the 1981 funding level. In addition, funds for the training of social service personnel were folded into the Title XX block grant—a measure which has the probable affect of reducing further the amount available to the states for actual social services. The Office of Management and Budgeting has estimated that in fiscal year 1981, approximately $575 million dollars or 21 percent of total program dollars had benefited elderly clients (U.S. Senate, 1982: 417). While states have wide discretion in deciding the type and amount of services made available under Title XX, the impact of the cutback noted can be expected to limit funds available for in-home and other community-based services for the frail elderly.

Also, a significant portion of social services funds under the Older Americans Act is spent on access, in-home, and legal services. The funding level for such services in fiscal year 1982 was at a $240.9 million level which represented a $10.56 million cut in funding over the previous year. In addition, combined funding for congregate meals and home delivered meals was reduced by almost $6 million dollars (U.S. Senate, 1982: 401). Such cutbacks further curtail the development and extension of in-home services and other related community-based services.

The cutbacks noted constitute a constraint on the impetus for developing an infrastructure of in-home and community-based services for the use of the frail elderly. Such fiscal constraint curtails the development on a national basis of a continuum of long-term care services having as a goal the maintenance of the chronically limited elderly in an environment which is "least restrictive" and most appropriate for the social and health needs of the individual.

SOME CONCLUDING COMMENTS

What is most needed in terms of Congressional consideration of provision of community-based services emphasizing home health and in-home social services is a bill which would present clear-cut comprehensive nationally defined areas of service (as did the Packwood Bill), and without necessarily medical dominance of the assessment process. Such a bill should statutorily determine a preadmission, screening, and assessment procedure which would allow for the determination of who can be most effectively cared for in the community, as well as assuring continuity of care in the least restrictive setting. Also, this bill should provide for a nationally mandated level of accessible services as well as statutorily mandated and federally implemented standards of care. National legislation should also provide a substantial commitment for resource development regarding home health and in-home social care. Finally, more encouragement is needed for direct family involvement in the home care of the frail elderly and other disabled individuals through significant tax credits or payments to family members, or other household caretakers, for homemaker and home health aide services rendered by such individuals to the frail elderly and other disabled individuals who would benefit from such community-based long-term care services.

Some cost advantages might accrue to such a community-based emphasis in terms of the reduction of less appropriate and more expensive hospital and nursing home stays. However, the main argument for such an emphasis on community-based care which allows the individual to function in an in-home setting should be more in the area of the appropriateness and effectiveness of community-based care, in terms of the social and physical health functioning of the frail elderly, as well as in maintaining the ideal of allowing such elderly persons to function in the least restrictive environment possible.

REFERENCES

H.R. 6194, 96th Cong., 2nd Sess.
Omnibus Reconciliation Act of 1980, *Conference Report,* 96th Cong., 2nd Sess., Report 96-1479.
Omnibus Budget Reconciliation Act of 1981, *Conference Report,* 97th Cong., 1st Sess., Report 97-208.
S.2809, 96th Cong., 2nd Sess.
S.234, 97th Cong., 1st Sess.
S.861, 97th Cong., 1st Sess.
U.S. Congress, Senate, Special Committee on Aging. *Developments on Aging, 1981,* Vol. 1, A Report of the Special Committee on Aging, 97th Cong., 2nd Sess., February 22, 1982.

SECTION IV

INTERNATIONAL POLICY CONSIDERATIONS REGARDING IN-HOME SERVICES FOR THE FRAIL ELDERLY

Chapter 8

In-Home Services for the Elderly: Some Comparative Examples

In Europe and in Canada, the late 1970s saw the rise of a trend to keep frail elderly people in their own homes and communities for as long as possible. This policy has resulted in a concern for providing in-home services and related supportive services that allow for the maintenance of the frail elderly (and the disabled) at home. In this chapter, we examine both the achievements and the organizational problems experienced in various national contexts.

Germany

One such experiment is the establishment of "sozialstationen" or home help centers in the Federal Republic of Germany. The aged constitute 70 percent to 90 percent of the clientele of such centers. By 1978, every state government in the Federal Republic of Germany had formulated a program for the reorganization of home care services within the concept of such community centers (Grunow, 1980: 312). Eighty-one such *sozialstationen* had developed within the various states. These centers are voluntary endeavors in which local governments participate financially and which also are subsidized by the various German states. Such *sozialstationen* are divided between "great" and "small" solutions of home care service delivery. The small solution primarily involves reorganization of services usually delivered by churches and voluntary organizations. The *sozialstationen* of such organizations offer home nursing services by a home or visiting nurse, home helps, and social helps for elderly persons. The great solution combines the aforementioned services with other therapeutic and social services. Such services would include social and psychological counseling.

The basic in-home services of the *sozialstationen* are home nursing care, "home helps," and homemaker services. Visiting nurse care would include personal care, washing, and bed making. The home nurse also can provide some technical care such as providing injections under a physician's order. Home helps provide aide with household chores, and may also provide personal aide including washing and household maintenance. Homemaker services which provide home help for the family is in effect "a substitute for the house wife" (Grunow, 1980:312-313). Grunow's research on services provided by 81 *sozialstationen* showed that nursing care and homemaker services were the core of community services for the elderly. Nursing care was delivered by all 81 centers while 68 provide homemaker services. Five centers provided additional chore services and home care aids. Additional social and health services provided by some of the 81 centers survey were[1]:

— meals on wheels	24
— referrals	19
— initiation of self-help in the neighborhood	14
— rental of home care appliances	14
— pedicure	9
— gymnastics, massages, baths	11
— mobile library, laundry service, visiting service, craftsmen service, etc.	9
— transportation service	7

Other services offered include the following[2]:

— counseling in everyday technical problems	21
— recreation services for the elderly	14
— psycho-social counseling	19
— ministerial services	3

Homemaker/home help service constitutes the key service provided by the *sozialstationen* system. This system has provided for the development of a common infrastructure furnishing social and

---

[1]Source: Dieter Grunow. " 'Sozialstationen' A New Model for Home Delivery of Care and Service." *The Gerontologist,* 20 (June 1980), 313.

[2]Source: Dieter Grunow. " 'Sozialistationen': A new Model for Home Delivery of Care and Service." *The Gerontologist,* 20 (June 1980), 313.

health care services and allowing an increasing number of the elderly to remain living at home for as long as they are able to do so.

Sweden

In Sweden, while old age nursing homes exist, public policy emphasizes home help services as a core service in an "open care" system—that is, a system of services that support elderly persons living in the community. Such home help services are combined with meal distribution, chiropody services, transportation and day care center services (Little, 1978: 283). Grants for such home-help services are provided by the central government in Sweden to defer 35 percent of a municipality's gross expenditures for the preceding year. Home help services provided under this system often include major components such as personal care, shopping, foot care, housekeeping, and the care of clothing. Responsibilities for home help services for the aged and the handicapped in Sweden is lodged in local authority social service departments. In a large city such as Stockholm, such access is provided at a district level. A resident of Stockholm lives in one of 17 social districts, each of which has a social services center.

Core home help services are provided for the elderly in every community. Other related services such as meals on wheels, chiropody, hairdressing, and bathing are also provided.

Because of a well developed infrastructure of welfare programs including income maintenance, rent subsidies, and health care services, special categorically related health and income programs for the elderly are not considered necessary. Home help services are generally free for persons whose main source of income is a governmental old age pension. Aged persons with higher incomes pay a fee scaled to their ability to pay. An exception is the case of health care, where nominal charges under the national health insurance system prevail. Home nursing services fall under the jurisdiction of the county councils and are implemented by district health authorities.

According to Little, the fact that matters pertaining to health and hospitals are under the jurisdiction of the Swedish county council may create a gap limiting coordination between home help and other social services of the personal social services system with the medical care delivery system (Little, 1978: 286-287). However, she goes on to note that at the level of in-home social services for the aged and handicapped program, coordination is excellent.

Denmark

In Denmark, most elderly live in their own homes or rented apartments, including publicly supported housing for the aged. Of individuals over age 65, only 6 percent live in nursing homes and only thirty-three percent of those 85 and over live in nursing homes (Friis, 1979: 204). According to the Danish Care Law, each municipality is obliged to establish a home health service with trained aides. Home helpers particularly utilized by the aged are permanent aids that provide assistance to persons who cannot perform domestic work due to frail health or permanent impairment. The work of home helpers includes "part time assistance with cleaning, washing, cooking, shopping, mending of clothes, personal hygiene, dressing and similar services" (Friis, 1979: 204). Home helpers are obliged since 1979 to take a program of studies consisting of a one week introductory course, followed by a four week basic course to be completed before the end of six months employment. This course includes an orientation in psychology, gerontology, social welfare, and health and social care for handicapped persons. To this program four supplementary courses are later added. Home nursing is offered by a separate home nurse service.

Home help services are free for persons with incomes which are not above the General Pension level. For those with incomes above this level, payments are graduated by income. About 25 percent of the households with one or more persons 70 years of age and over receive home help. Seventy-five percent of households receive 1 to 6 hours help per week, 18 percent receive 7 to 12 hours weekly aid, and 7 percent receive over 12 hours weekly (Friis, 1979: 205).

Municipalities are planning an increase in the number of home helpers and plan extensions of home help service to include evening and weekend services. All municipalities must also provide free nursing service upon physician referral. Home nurses execute treatment prescribed by physicians and provide additional nursing care. In more than half of Denmark's municipalities the home nurse is supervised by a supervisory home nurse. Home nurses coordinate their activities with hospitals, general practitioners and home helpers. Often municipalities provide planned coordination of home nurse and home helper services through a joint executive committee of both services or through municipal home care centers. About 15 percent of persons 65 or older received home health care in 1977 (Friis, 1979: 205).

In addition to in-home social care and nursing services under Denmark's Care Law, municipalities provide a number of avenues of assistance to elderly persons (and others) with permanent functional limitations. Municipalities may make technical alterations in dwellings such as the removal of doorsteps, kitchen alterations, and installation of banisters so that they improve a person's ability to remain at home. Municipalities may provide wheelchairs, artificial limbs, hearing aids, and glasses as well as telephones and specially designed household equipment. They also have established day care homes for elderly people with major needs whose relatives look after them after working hours. Transportation to such homes is provided. Day care centers also are provided. Centers deliver such services as chiropody, physiotherapy and recreation. To a lesser extent, home visiting and meals-on-wheels services are provided by voluntary groups and municipalities.

Friis notes that the network of home services for the aged has not interfered with the continuing relationship of the elderly with their children. A survey by the National Institute for Social Research in 1977 observes that:

> 11 percent of those 62 years and over who had a child were living with a child, of those living alone or with a spouse, 38 percent had seen a child at the day of the interview or the day before and 32 percent had seen a child 2-7 days before; well over half of the aged received various kinds of assistance from their children. (Friis, 1979: 206)

Denmark presents an example of a national policy of community care for the elderly and other functionally limited persons focused on in-home social and health services implemented at the municipal level. The municipalities make a conscious effort to coordinate home help and home health services. This emphasis does not impede—rather it appears to enhance continued family support by children of elderly persons.

Canada

A fourth structure of provision of home care is provided by Canada (Gommer, Hankenne, and Rogowski, 1979: 128-129). Home care and home nursing are closely tied to the health care system in Canada's provinces. When a decision is made within the hospital that a frail elderly (or other ill) patient may continue his treatment at home, a home liaison nurse, the hospital nurse, and the case physician determine, in consultation, whether home conditions allow for such care. After a decision to proceed with home care, the nurses train the patient and his family in nursing techniques and hygiene areas—principal components of a home care program. Home care organizations in Canada are privately run and totally governmentally subsidized—as a matter of national governmental policy. Home help services including baths, house cleaning, and the preparation of meals are limited to the acutely ill elderly—in part because of the limited number of available trained personnel.

CONCLUSION

Patterns of community care for the elderly have as their core home care services. Such services are not solely provided to the elderly—however, the elderly are a primary target group for such services. Increasingly, as a matter of public policy, a number of "developed" nations seek to maintain the frail elderly in their own homes and out of institutions for as long as is possible. The main issues faced by such systems of services are (1) integration of a network of community-based care services having as its core home care services for the frail aged, and (2) whether the integration of personal care services is coordinated with necessary health services. Other issues discussed are the degree of linkage between national government policy and delivery of service by local or provincial government or by voluntary auspices funded by such local or provincial governments.

REFERENCES

Friis, Henning. "The Aged in Denmark: Social Programmes," pp. 201-211 in *Reaching the Aged: Social Services in Forty-Four Countries*, edited by Morton I. Teicher, Daniel Thursz, and Joseph L. Viglante. Beverly Hills/London: Sage Publications, 1979.
Gommers, Adrienne; Hankenne, Bernadette; and Rogowski, Beatrice. "Help Structures for the Aged: Experience in Seven Countries," pp. 117-145, in *Reaching the Aged: Social Services in Forty-Four Countries*, edited by Morton I. Teicher, Daniel Thursz, and Joseph L. Vigilante. Beverly Hills/London: Sage Publications, 1979.
Grunow, Deiter, "Sozialstationen? A New Model for Home Delivery of Care and Service." *The Gerontologist*, 20 (June 1980), 308-317.
Little, Virginia. "Open Care for the Aged: Swedish Model." *Social Work*, 23 (July 1978), 282-287.

Afterword:
Some Conclusions

Currently no articulated, well-formulated national policy exists attempting to meet the needs of many of our frail elderly citizens in a manner commensurate with their living in a non-institutional, at-home setting. Nor does a policy exist which seeks at a national level to involve and support family and friends with respect to meeting the home health and home social care needs and other community-based service needs of the frail and functionally limited elderly. Also lacking is a national information-gathering and reporting system which could provide an informed basis for the development of national policy in this important area. Many of the home health, home social care and other community-based programs which do exist are matters of state or local option. This leads to a great deal of inequity between regions in the meeting of community-based health and social care service needs of the functionally limited elderly. In many areas, needed in-home services are so unavailable that such services are visibly inadequate in terms of meeting the needs of the frail elderly. Also, existing long-term care programs are often inadequate because they do not sufficiently emphasize the need for community-based and in-home care; they do not sufficiently emphasize the health and social care needs of elderly persons with chronic, long-term limitations, and they do not sufficiently take into account the family unit. In the one program that is a truly national program, Medicare home health services, the requirement that services be related to an acute medical condition ignores the functional needs of many elderly persons for in-home homemaker/home aide care on a continuing basis. Also, the vendor payment basis of Medicare services results in many inequities between regions regarding the presence of available levels of in-home health service, the quality of such services, and the comprehensiveness of such services.

In the viewpoint of the authors, the moral fiber of a civilized society is reflected in the care with which it treats its most vulnerable populations—children, the disabled, and the frail elderly. A number of European countries have as a basis of policy towards their elder citizens set the goal of maintaining them in an in-home setting as long as this is an appropriate setting. They have provided services aimed at fulfilling that policy goal. The role of family members in such care is often a conscious element in the development of such national policies.

We have, we believe, demonstrated the need for such nationally developed policies and programs. We also have shown the shortcomings of the incremental, fragmented, and uncoordinated programs which are the legacy of the 1970s.